Chinese Auricular Acupuncture

Chinese Auricular Acupuncture

SKYA ABBATE

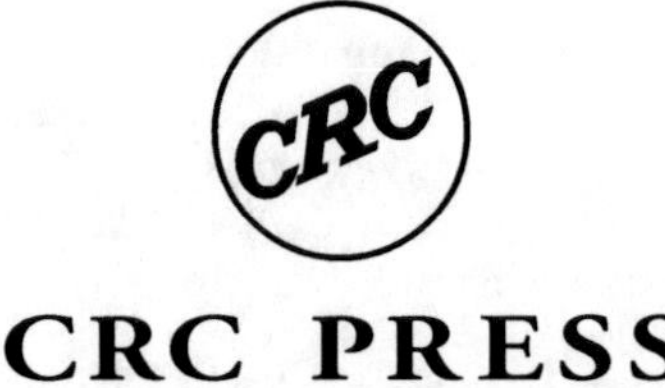

CRC PRESS

Boca Raton London New York Washington, D.C.

Photographs by David A. Brown and Anthony Abbate
Calligraphy by Dr. Jishun Hao, DOM
Illustrations by Jaye Oliver

Medical knowledge is constantly changing. As new information becomes available, changes in treatment, procedures, equipment and the use of drugs become necessary. The author and the publisher have taken care to ensure that the information given in this text is accurate and up to date. However, readers are strongly advised to confirm that the information complies with the latest legislation and standards of practice. It is recommended that patients be under the care of a licensed healthcare provider.

Library of Congress Cataloging-in-Publication Data

Abbate, Skya.
Chinese auricular acupuncture / Skya Abbate.
p. cm.
Includes bibliographical references and index.
Contents: The ear: an ancient microsystem with modern applications — The anatomical terminology of auricular medicine — The location of 100 common ear points — The clinical energetics of the ear points — Cautions and contraindications — Ear modalities — Ear diagnosis and morphology — Ear prescription construction and formulas for specific conditions — Clinical research and effective points.
ISBN 0-8493-2052-6 (alk. paper)
1. Ear—Acupuncture. I. Title.

RM184.A234 2003
615.8′92—dc21 2003055166

Direct all inquiries to CRC Press LLC, 2000 N.W. Corporate Blvd., Boca Raton, Florida 33431.

International Standard Book Number 0-8493-2052-6
Library of Congress Card Number 2003055166
Printed in the United States of America 2 3 4 5 6 7 8 9 0
Printed on acid-free paper

Dedication

To my nephews and nieces: Anthony, Mark, Jennifer, Alex, Lauren, Rebekah, Elizabeth, Laura Grace, Nicole, Leah, David, Aaron, Adam, and Seth

Remember — All good things are possible with God

Foreword

Pursuing an integrated approach to treatment, the practitioner of Chinese medicine must hold a clinical view that extends from a patient's depth to the outermost branch of his or her physical being. The practitioner must be able to touch the aspect of being that, in the context of the moment, will most efficiently help to promote functional balance. Skya Abbate has furthered the ability of practitioners to achieve these ideals by providing a comprehensive survey of ear acupuncture.

Skya's text has the potential to allow the diligent reader to fully integrate treatment of the ear into clinical practice. Based on her many years of study and clinical experience, she illustrates for us the aspects of auricular therapy that she has found to be most effective. But more importantly, she provides a substantial foundation so we can continue to expand our knowledge of auricular therapy as we gain clinical experience.

Her inclusion of a detailed section on ear diagnosis will allow readers to supplement their assessment of the pulse, tongue, and hara, thus improving our ability to differentiate the functional basis of imbalance and illness. Unlike so many other texts, the ear is not presented as a "black box" whose efficacy is based on some mysterious cause-and-effect relationship to symptoms. Rather than merely provide a list of points and symptoms for the practitioner to learn by rote, Skya explains the theory behind ear treatment in a way that is consistent with Chinese physiology. Her detailed tables and photographs serve as clear aids to help the student grasp whatever point she is illustrating.

Having read *Chinese Auricular Acupuncture*, I was inspired to integrate auricular therapy and diagnosis into my own clinical practice, and I have been very pleased with the results. Skya's book is a gift to any practitioner wishing to extend his or her diagnostic abilities and clinical effectiveness.

Lonny S. Jarrett, M.Ac.,
Author of *Nourishing Destiny: The Inner Tradition of Chinese Medicine*

Preface

The purpose of this book is to provide students and practitioners of Oriental medicine with a clear, concise, user-friendly manual on ear acupuncture. Many books abound on this topic, yet in this author's experience, they tend to make the study of the ear more complicated than it needs to be. Additionally, most are not practically oriented for the student or clinician who is interested in an easy to do, yet efficacious, modality. Nor do such books tend to explain auricular medicine within the framework of traditional Oriental energetics that is consistent with the use of the medicine. In this text, the reader is given the opportunity to reduce the need for memorization or the need to consult manuals for reference because the method of using ear acupuncture is consonant with the underpinnings of an education in traditional Chinese medicine.

I have practiced ear acupuncture for over 20 years and have taught it for over a decade. This adds to my ability to deliver a manual that can be studied independently and then easily used to treat the many diseases that characterize the human condition. But ultimately, the simplicity of the paradigm presented and the way it is exposed should allow the reader to see the practical utilization of auricular therapy within the practice of Oriental medicine. In this way one can be weaned from the text because the thought processes of how to locate points, select modalities, construct prescriptions, and apply them to the uniqueness of each person have been carefully organized and outlined. In contrast to many books, only one ear map is referred to instead of pages and pages of maps and systems. Thus, the art of auricular medicine is elegantly simplified.

In addition to this central focus, this book contains other features that distinguish it from comparable texts. Differentiating features include the following:

- Many photos of actual ears illustrate the pathology commonly seen in the ear. This pathology is incorporated into the text in order to teach differentiating ear morphology and diagnosis.
- Most ear modalities (such as needles, press tacks, seeds, etc.) are also pictured to demonstrate treatment tools with which the practitioner may be unfamiliar, but might want to learn.

- Actual cases from clinical practice are incorporated to illustrate the clinical applicability of specific modalities and ear acupuncture points.
- The clinical energetics of the ear points are described in classical Chinese medical terms, so that the practitioner can ascertain how to select ear acupuncture points to correspond with the most common Chinese diagnostic paradigms.
- An extensive bibliography covering close to 800 books and journals written over a 30-year period is included and summarized in pertinent places throughout the book.
- A discussion of how to construct ear acupuncture prescriptions is offered and analyzed, so that the practitioner can learn how to construct his own prescriptions and not be dependent upon any text, including this one.
- Many prescriptions that I have devised for specific clinical populations are presented and dissected in order to teach the practitioner the thought processes behind ear acupuncture prescription writing. Formulae derived from two internships I did in China are also listed and analyzed for similar purposes.

In conclusion, the greatest strength of this book is its user-friendliness, which equally allows both the beginning student and the experienced practitioner to successfully apply auricular medicine in the treatment of their patients in a caring, relatively noninvasive, and effective manner.

Skya Abbate
Southwest Acupuncture College

Acknowledgments

To the students of Southwest Acupuncture College, Santa Fe, New Mexico, for "lending me their ears" while they let me teach this material to them for the past 13 years.

To Thomas Martinez, for his expert computer skills in preparing most of the tables for this book.

To Stuart Watts, who as my first teacher and practitioner, taught me the inestimable power of ear acupuncture.

To my husband, Anthony, for always believing in me.

About the Author

Skya Abbate, M.A., D.O.M., Dipl.Ac., Dipl. C.H., began her career as a medical sociologist serving as a Peace Corps volunteer in Brazil, and later taught in the sociology department of the University of Rhode Island (1978 to 1981). She holds a bachelor of arts in sociology from Salve Regina College, Newport, Rhode Island (1973), where she graduated summa cum laude and as class valedictorian. Abbate earned her master of arts in sociology from the University of Rhode Island (1978), during which time she worked as the manager of the Alternative Food Co-op at URI as well as pursuing premed studies at the same university.

In 1983, Skya graduated from the acupuncture program of the Institute of Traditional Medicine, Santa Fe, New Mexico. She undertook two advanced clinical training programs with the Academy of Traditional Chinese Medicine in Beijing, China (1988, 1989).

A licensed doctor of Oriental medicine in the state of New Mexico and executive director of Southwest Acupuncture College (with campuses in Santa Fe and Albuquerque, New Mexico and Boulder, Colorado), Skya was former president of the New Mexico Association of Acupuncture and Oriental Medicine. She has served over 6 years as an educational expert and commissioner for the Accreditation Commission for Acupuncture and Oriental Medicine, the national organization that accredits professional degree programs in Oriental medicine.

Skya is the author of three additional books — *Beijing: The New Forbidden City* (Southwest Acupuncture College Press, 1991), *Holding the Tiger's Tail: An Acupuncture Techniques Manual in the Treatment of Disease* (Southwest Acupuncture College Press, 1996), and *The Art of Palpatory Diagnosis in Oriental Medicine* (Churchill Livingstone, 2001). She is also the author of over 30 journal articles in the *American Journal of Acupuncture,* the *Journal of Chinese Medicine*, the *New England Journal of Traditional Chinese Medicine*, and *Acupuncture Today,* a monthly American newsletter, in which she is now in her fourth year of writing as the needle technique columnist. Two new texts are in progress — *The Spiritual Practice of Clinical Medicine* and a point location and energetics book, along with a book of poetry and numerous Catholic inspirational short stories.

Skya teaches needle technique, diagnosis, and Japanese acupuncture systems at Southwest Acupuncture College in New Mexico. She also has a private practice integrating classical Chinese treatment with her subspecialty in Japanese acupuncture.

Contents

chapter one

The ear: an ancient microsystem with modern applications

Objectives

- To gain a sense of the history and development of ear acupuncture
- To learn the applicability of auricular medicine to the treatment of many conditions

Introduction

Embedded within the rigid curves of the external ear are the powerful ear acupuncture points that correspond to every part of the body. This incredible organ, the first of all our organs to develop embryologically, is not only the vehicle for the perception of sound and, thereby, our connection with fellow humans and the larger environment, but it is also an instrument that fulfills several other equally astonishing functions in the realm of medicine. Whether small or delicate, normal or large in size and shape, traditional Chinese medicine demonstrates that the ear is an extraordinarily powerful nexus of energy through which the entire body can be treated because all of the organs and body parts are represented within its concentric folds. This configuration makes it a complete microsystem for the treatment of many human illnesses.

Although most acupuncture practitioners are well aware of the system of ear medicine as a highly effective method for treating illness, perhaps they are less familiar with the power of the ear as a diagnostic tool for the detection of an existing illness, be it musculoskeletal, organ related or even emotional in nature, or the possible perception of one's genetic predispositions. This fascinating feature of auricular medicine, a direct product of the reflexive nature of the ear as a microsystem, provides valuable medical insight into the health of the whole person. Thus, not only are diagnosis and treatment accomplished through ear acupuncture medicine, but also numerous health disorders can be prevented through the discernment of the pathology appearing on the surface of the auricle when it is correctly detected and correspondingly treated. Auricular medicine is versatile as well, allowing ear treatment to be used successfully either as an independent therapy or in combination with other therapeutic modalities so as to reinforce the outcome of treatment.

History

In Oriental medical literature, numerous Chinese texts refer to the role of the ear as an instrument for the diagnosis, prognosis, prevention, and treatment of disease. Most of these texts go back to the earliest recorded Chinese body of medical information, wherein they established the connection between the ear and all of the meridians, the *Zang-fu* organs, and the Kidney in particular because the ear is its external manifestation. One such reference from the oldest extant Chinese text, the *Neijing (The Yellow Emperor's Classic of Internal Medicine,* 500 to 300 B.C.) included the observation that the ear is not an isolated organ, but intimately connected with all the organs of the body, the five viscera, and the six bowels.[1] In the Oral inquiry chapter of the *Mystical Gate,* it states that the ear is the converging place of the main vessels. Because the ear is connected to every part of the body due to the ceaseless circulation of air and blood through these meridians and vessels, the ear joins with the body to form a unified inseparable whole.[2] Later in the *Zhongcangjing (The Classic of Central Organs)* from the Sung Dynasty (920 to 1279 A.D.) it was written that prognosis could be judged from inspection of the auricle.[3]

Despite the early mention in Chinese medical literature of the connection of the ear to the rest of the body, it was not until 1957, under the careful aegis of noted French acupuncturist Paul Nogier, that a system of auricular medicine was formalized. Up to that point even the Chinese had not published a chart of ear points. In his book, the *Treatise of Auriculotherapy,* Nogier established the correspondences between the sensitive points in the auricle and the internal organs of the body and expounded his view that the points on the auricle were organized in the form of a homunculus very similar to an inverted fetus, with the head towards the lower lobule, the feet towards the upper rim of the ear, and the body in-between.

Terry Oleson, commenting on Nogier's pioneer work said, "It is believed that it was through this German publication that Nogier's inverted fetus map of the ear was ultimately translated into Chinese and formed the basis of Chinese ear charts. However, once presented with this concept, the Chinese conducted thorough and systematic investigations. Both the diagnostic accuracy and therapeutic value of the inverted fetus ear map were examined in over 2000 clinical cases by the Nanking Army Ear Acupuncture team. They provided significant verification of the somatotopic conceptualization of the ear and discovered some additional points not noted in Nogier's auricular charts."[4] It thus was Nogier who elevated ear acupuncture in status within the field of Oriental medicine, for as ear researcher Michael Greenwood so eloquently summarizes, "In a stroke, Nogier transformed ear acupuncture from an esoteric field into a simple and powerful modality."[5]

Since then, various leaders in the field of Oriental medicine have created other ear charts. The chart presented by Bensky and O'Connor in *Acupuncture, A Comprehensive Text* depicts more points than the chart presented in this book. Nogier and the European schools discuss different locations of the points based on various physiological states they may assume. Oleson's approach is more anatomical. Likewise, he uses the nervous system as the major explanation for how ear points work and the nomenclature of many of his points varies as well.

All of these sources are impeccable and can be consulted for added information about the ear. However, because I have learned another system and have practiced it exclusively with great success for 20 years, these sources are neither part of my clinical experience nor my philosophical predilection as a practitioner of Oriental medicine. Hence, in this book, I cannot reconcile their differences nor expound knowledgeably upon them for the reader.

The map that forms the basis of the location of the ear acupuncture point system presented in this book comes from the scheme of ear point location taught to me by the doctors with whom I studied at the International Training Center of the Academy of Traditional Chinese Medicine in Beijing, China in 1988 and 1989. It is one chart, almost identical to the ear chart found in *Chinese Acupuncture and Moxibustion,* the primary textbook from China that is used in almost all acupuncture schools throughout the U.S. and beyond. This chart has been the same since the 1980s when the first version of the book was published. Simply organized, the chart encompasses most body parts and organ systems and, as such, it can be used to treat every condition treatable through the ear with great results.

Of these points, for purposes of simplicity and the clinical frequency with which these points are chosen, I am presenting 100 points with their locations and most common clinical functions. The strength of the 100 points of the Chinese ear map that I have adopted and the energetic or physiological actions that pertain to them, is that they are easy to learn and use, and can be used to treat every condition that is relevant to the application of auricular medicine. They can be mastered easily, especially if one has strong training in the theoretical infrastructure of Oriental medicine.

Anatomy and physiology of the ear

The ability of the ear to evoke the dramatic changes that it does can be linked to its unique Oriental physiological energetics. The historical references cited at the beginning of this chapter provide some of the physiological rationales for the mechanisms of ear acupuncture. A review of the internal and external pathways of the 12 *Zang-fu* organs also reveals this connection.

According to Western anatomy, the ear as a whole is composed of elastic cartilage, fat, and connective tissue. This composition, in its healthy state, causes the ear to feel both firm yet flexible instead of too soft, brittle, or rigid. Because of these normal characteristics, when the ear is palpated in the physical examination, anything other than firmness and flexibility is regarded as pathological.

From a Western viewpoint and for those who use such an orientation, the nervous innervations of the ear are the leading explanation of how and why auricular therapy works. Essentially, the nerves that innervate the ear have connections with the internal organs and all parts of the body. Many researchers such as W. E. Spoerel, deduce the "needling of effective loci and particularly ear needling often causes an instantaneous reduction or disappearance of pain; the speed of this response can only be explained by a mechanism within the nervous system."[6]

Such nervous innervations are highly complex and for purposes of much auriculotherapy formatted from an Oriental viewpoint and expressed in this book, it is not necessary to know the names of the nerves and which ear points they innervate because, in the system of Chinese ear acupuncture, the mechanism for how it works is primarily explained through the meridian system. The reader can consult Western textbooks on this subject as well as many of the books listed in the bibliography if neurological pathways are an area of further interest.

Some authors have advanced the theory that the close proximity of the ear to the brain and, thus, the likelihood of nervous mediation, is the reason auriculoacupoints work so well. Peter Hubner writes that "at precisely the same time in embryological development when the spinal cord is forming (within the first 8 to 12 days of mesodermal unfolding), a knob develops within the brain that ultimately becomes the external ear."[7] This fact illustrates the close relationship between the ear, the brain, and the nervous system. Hubner also points out that the ear is the first organ to develop to its full size and becomes fully functional approximately 18 weeks after conception. It is also the first sensory organ to begin working as early as the 8th week *in utero*.

The ear is richly supplied with blood vessels. All of the arteries supplying the auricle come from the external carotid artery. This dense vascularization of the ear makes the helix of the ear reddish in hue and the ear warm. These are normal features found during inspection of the ear. According to medical acupuncturist Joseph Helms, "The vasculature at the auricular points is compressed and more tightly intertwined with myelinated nerve fibers than in the body points."[8] This combination of vascularization and nerve innervations in the ear accounts for the strong stimulus obtained in ear acupuncture as well as its faster rate of reactivity compared with body acupuncture points, and thus its valuable clinical utility as a site for treatment.

The ear is more susceptible to infection than other body parts because it is replete with lymphatic vessels that drain into several nodes in the area of the neck. This anatomical fact is important to keep in mind when treating the ear so that infection does not develop or spread. This can be achieved by observing strict aesepsis of the ear.

In summary, both these Western and Chinese anatomical facts and physiological theories offer reasons for the therapeutic effectiveness of the auricle as a site for treatment, and they are not antithetical to each other. Their theories explain, for instance, why effective auricular treatment typically produces a sensation of heat (due to vascularization). The Western categorization of the ear as connective tissue, which is essentially elastic cartilage, and the Chinese notion that healthy ears are supple and not stiff or brittle, are also perfect correspondences.

The clinical utility of the ear for diagnosis, treatment, and prevention

Ear acupuncture is very effective for those illnesses that are within the realm of Oriental medicine to treat, both with body acupuncture and herbs. In over 20 years of clinical experience, I have found that the therapeutic effectiveness of ear acupuncture is in the 90% range and this scope covers a broad spectrum of diseases. Disorders that are most treatable with ear acupuncture include musculoskeletal problems, such as knee, shoulder, and ankle problems; hormonal disorders, such as hot flashes associated with menopause; thyroid disorders and menstrual problems; and diseases of the *Zang-fu* organs, such as stomach ulcers, asthma and allergies, and digestive problems, just to name a few. Specifically, the ear is an excellent site to treat any problem that has a pain component, such as low back pain, migraines, skin disorders (i.e., dermatitis), and neurological and vascular problems, such as multiple sclerosis and high blood pressure, respectively. Emotional problems, such as anxiety, also are treated satisfactorily through this method.

Nogier claims that ear acupuncture has four major usages. He purports that the best indication of auriculotherapy is the presence of pain, including extreme cancer pain. Also, it is useful in the treatment of painful shingles if caught early. It can be employed for emotional problems involving the central nervous system. It makes patients more sensitive to drug therapy by changing metabolism thereby increasing absorption and elimination, and it can be used to effectively treat addictions.[9] I found all of these claims to be true as well.

Apart from its clinical efficacy, historical roots, and contemporary usage, there are other features that make employing ear acupuncture a valuable option. They include the following:

- Auricular medicine is easy to learn and master.
- Ear acupuncture tools are not costly. Regardless of which modality (needles, pellets, etc.) is selected for treatment, the equipment required for ear acupuncture is minimal and relatively inexpensive.
- Ear acupuncture can be used as an exclusive and independent modality, or as an adjunct to therapy that serves to enhance the treatment initiated through the other methods.

- The results obtained from auriculoacupuncture are quick, effective, and time-tested with over a 2500-year history.
- Ear acupuncture is a relatively noninvasive technique that is both convenient to the patient in terms of ease of administration and promotes the patient's compliance through self-treatment.
- Unless it is used inappropriately, ear acupuncture incurs no negative side effects.
- Auricular medicine has a broad range of applicability to numerous clinical conditions, including the diagnosis, treatment, and prevention of disease.
- Like body acupuncture, ear acupuncture can be used for the treatment of diseases of the internal organs, musculoskeletal, and emotional problems. Ear therapy is particularly effective for the treatment of pain, inflammation, and skin disorders, and can treat both acute and chronic disease.
- The ear can be used successfully for virtually every clinical condition, producing at least a 90% success rate.
- Like body acupuncture, if properly applied, the strength of auricular acupuncture is that it stimulates the body to heal itself according to the principles of balancing *Yin* and *Yang* and promoting proper organ function. Helmut Kropej reminds us though, "… regardless of the specific illness with which you are dealing, you must always keep the pathophysiological cause in mind. Only then will you be able to get to the root of the disorder."[10]

We must keep these factors in mind when we construct ear acupuncture prescriptions and proceed to treatment.

References

1. Huang, H. *Ear Acupuncture*. Rodale Press, Emmaus, PA, 1974, p. 1.
2. Ibid, p. 3.
3. *Practical Ear Needling*, 3rd ed. Medicine and Health Publishing Company, Hong Kong, September 1982, p. 1.
4. Oleson, T. and Kroening, R. A comparison of Chinese and Nogier auricular acupuncture points. *Am. J. Acupunc.*, 1983 (July–September), 11(3): 206.
5. Greenwood, M. The use of ear acupuncture to promote vaginal delivery after Cesarean section. *Am. J. Acupunc.*, 1992, 20(4): 308.
6. Spoerel, W.E., Varkey, M., and Leung, C. Acupuncture in chronic pain. *Am. J. Chin. Med.*, 1976 Autumn; 4(3): 267–279.
7. Hubner, P., *The Special Status of the Ear in Organism*, Medical Resonance Therapy Music®, Digital Pharmacy, AAR Edition International, 2001.
8. Helms, J. *Acupuncture Energetics: A Clinical Approach for Physicians*. Medical Acupuncture Publishers, Berkeley, CA, 1995, p. 136.
9. Nogier, P. *Handbook of Auriculotherapy*. Maisonneuve, Moulins-les-Metz, France, 1981, p. 119.

10. Kropej, H. *The Fundamentals of Ear Acupuncture,* 4th ed. Karl F. Haug Publishers, Heidelberg, Germany, 1991, p. 31.

Bibliography

Barskii, V.D. Reflexotherapy of vibration-induced disease. *ZH Nevropatol. Psikhiatr. Im. S.S. Korsakova,* 1988, 88(4): 65–68, (in Russian).

Biedebach, M. Accelerated healing of skin ulcers by electrical stimulation and the intracellular physiological mechanisms involved. *Am. J. Acupunc. (Abs.),* 1989 4: 103.

Borozan, S. and Petkovie, G. Ear acupuncture has a hypotonic effect on the gastrointestinal tract. *Vojnosanit. Pregl.,* Jan.–Feb. 1996, 53(1): 31–33, (in Serbo–Croatian).

Bragin, E.O. Alteration of opiate-like substance content in auricular electroacupuncture analgesia of rats. *Voprosy. Medit. Khimii.,* 1982, 28 (4): 102–105, (in Russian).

Bragin, E.O., Batueva, N.N., and Durinian, R.A. Role of the somatic monoaminergic systems in the mechanisms of regulation of pain sensitivity during reflex stimulation. *Biull. Eksp. Biol. Med.,* Oct. 1983, 96(10): 9–12, (in Russian).

Bragin, E.O., Batueva, N.N., and Monaenkov, K.A. Role of catecholamine neurons in the reticular lateral nuclei in regulating sensitivity to pain during exposure to reflex stimuli. *Biull. Eksp. Biol. Med.,* May 1983, 95(5): 119–121, (in Russian).

Bragin, E.O., Batueva, N.N., and Vasilenko, G.F. Role of giant cell nuclei of the reticular formation in mechanisms of analgesia during auricular electroacupuncture and action of morphine. *Biull. Eksp. Biol. Med.,* Oct. 1988, 106(12): 390–392, (in Russian).

Bragin, E.O., Vasilenko, G.F., and Durinjan, R.A. The study of the central grey matter in mechanisms of different kinds of analgesia: effects of lesions. *Pain,* May 1983, 16(1): 33–40.

Bresler, D.E., Cohen, J.S., Kroening, R., Levin, N., and Sadoff, A. The potential of acupuncture for the behavioral sciences. *Am. Psychol.,* Mar. 1975, 30(3): 411–414.

Ceccherelli, F., Altafini, L., Varotto, E., and Stefecius, A. The effect of benzodiazepines administration on auricular symptomatological evidence. *Acupunc. Electrother. Res.,* 1990, 115(2): 95–106.

Chaitow, L. *The Acupuncture Treatment of Pain.* Healing Arts Press, Rochester, VT, 1990.

Chan, P. *Ear Acupressure: Healing and Treating Pain by the Therapeutic Stimulation of Acupuncture Points in the Ear by Use of Finger Pressure.* Thorsens, London, 1981.

Chen, B.Y. Acupuncture normalizes dysfunction of hypothalamic–pituitary–ovarian axis. *Acupunc. Electrother. Res.,* 1997, 22: 97–108.

Chen, C.J. and Yu, H.S. Acupuncture treatment of urticaria. *Arch. Dermatol.,* Nov. 1998, 134(11): 1397–1399.

Chen, H. Recent studies on auriculoacupuncture and its mechanism. *J. Trad. Chin. Med.,* June 1993, 13(2): 129–143.

Chen, L., Liu, X., Wang, X., Yan, G., Hao, X., Wang, L., and Mu, Y. Effects of ear acupuncture on beta-adrenoreceptor in lung tissues of guinea pigs with experimental asthma. *Zhen Ci Yan Jiu,* 1996, 21(1): 56–59, (in Chinese).

Chien, C.H., Sjieh, J.Y., Laio, M.H., Ling, E.A., and Wen, C.Y. Neuronal connections between the sympathetic pre– and postganglionic neurons of the dog as studied by using pseudo rabies virus. *Neurosci. Res., 1998,* 30: 169–175.

Cotton, R.T. The ear, nose, oropharynx, and larynx, in *Rudolph's Pediatrics,* Rudolph, A.M., Hoffman, J.I.E., and Rudolph, C.D., Eds., Appelton–Lange, Stamford, CT, 1996, p. 945.

Dale, R.A. Systems, holograms, and theory of micro-acupuncture. *Am. J. Acupunc.,* 1999, 27(3–4): 207–242.

Dung, H.C. Role of the vagus nerve in weight reduction through auricular acupuncture. *Am. J. Acupunc.,* 1986, 14(3): 249–254.

Greenwood, M. The use of ear acupuncture to promote vaginal delivery after cesarean section. *Am. J. Acupunc.,* 1992, 20(4): 308–312.

Haker, E., Egekvist, H., and Bjerring, P. Effect of sensory stimulation (acupuncture) on sympathetic and parasympathetic activities in healthy subjects. *J. Auton. Nerv. Syst.,* Feb. 14, 2000, 79(1): 520–529.

Helms, J. *Acupuncture Energetics: A Clinical Approach for Physicians.* Medical Acupuncture Publishers, Berkeley, CA, 1995.

Ho, W.K., Wen, H.L., Lam, S., and Ma, L. The influence of electro-acupuncture on naloxone-induced morphine withdrawal in mice: elevation of brain opiate-like activity. *Eur. J. Pharmacol.,* May 15, 1978, 49(2): 197–199

Hu, R. Basic research on auricular acupuncture. *Zhong Xi Yi He Za Zhi,* Jun. 1990, 10(6): 379–82, (in Chinese).

Huang, H. *Ear Acupuncture.* Rodale Press, Emmaus, PA, 1974.

Ishibashi, S. The effect of auricular acupuncture on the neuronal activity of the thalamic and hypothalamic neurons of the rat. *Acupunc. Electrother. Res.,* 1986, 11(1): 15–23.

Kajdos, V. Experiences with auricular acupuncture. *Am. J. Acupunc.,* 1976, 4(2): 130–136.

Kangmei, C., Shulian, Z., and Ying, Z. Clinical application of traditional auriculotherapy (continued). *J. Trad. Chin. Med.,* 1993, 13: 152–154.

Kawakita, K., Kawamura, H., Keino, H., Hongo, T., and Kitakohji, H. Development of the low impedance points in the auricular skin of experimental peritonitis rats. *Am. J. Chin. Med.,* 1991, 19(3–4): 199–205.

Kho, H.G., Van Egmond, J., Eijk, R.J., and Kapteyns, W.M. Lack of influence of acupuncture and transcutaneous stimulation on the immunoglobulin levels and leukocyte counts following upper-abdominal surgery. *Eur. J. Anaesthesiol.,* Jan. 1991, 8(1): 39–45.

Khrqamov, R.N., Karpuk, N.I., Vorob'ev, V.V., Gal'chenko, A.A., and Kosarshii, L.S. The electrical activity of the hypothalamus in exposure to millimeter-wave radiation at biologically active points. *Biull. Eksp. Biol. Med.,* Sept. 1993, 116: 263–265, (in Russian).

Kitade, T. and Hyodo, M. The effects of stimulation of ear acupuncture points on the body's pain threshold. *Am. J. Chin. Med.,* 1979, 7(3): 241–252.

Kitade, T., et al. The meridian phenomenon induced by ear acupuncture in a meridian-sensitive patient. *J. Jpn. Soc. Acupunc. Moxi.,* 1984, 33(3): 298–302.

Kozma, A. Auriculotherapy: a method for inducing analgesia in the stomatological practice. *Rev. Chir. Oncol. O. R. L. Oftalmol. Ser. Stomatol.,* Apr.–Jun. 1987, 34(2): 139–149, (in Romanian).

Kropej, H. *The Fundamentals of Ear Acupuncture, 4th ed.,* Karl F. Haug Publishers, Heidelberg, Germany, 1991.

Lein, D. et al. Comparison of effect of transcutaneous electrical nerve stimulation of auricular and somatic, and the combination of auricular and somatic acupuncture points in experimental threshold. *Phys. Ther.*, Aug. 1989, 69: 6717–6718.

Liu, S. *Auricular Diagnosis, Treatment, and Health Preservation.* Science Press, Beijing, China, 1996.

Liu, Y. and Minkov, M. The external ear/embryo relationship explains the basis of ear acupuncture. *Pac. J. Orient. Med.*, Mar. 1999, 7: 20–23.

Lu, H.C. *A Complete Textbook of Auricular Acupuncture, 2nd ed.* The Academy of Oriental Heritage, Vancouver B.C., Canada, 1975.

Medicine and Health Publishing Co., *Practical Ear Needling, 3rd ed.* Hong Kong, Sept. 1982.

Meizerov, E.E., Reshetniak, V.K., and Durinian, R.A. Reflex suppression of evoked nocioceptive responses in the parafasicular complex and posterior ventromedial nucleus of the thalamus in cats during electroacupuncture. *Biull. Eksp. Biol. Med.*, Aug. 1981, 92(8): 12–14, (in Russian).

Moskovets, O.N. Effect of auricular acupuncture on the motor manifestations of nocioceptive reactions. *Biull. Eksp. Biol. Med.*, Apr. 1980, 89(4): 401–403, (in Russian).

Moskovets, O.N., Reshetniak, V.K., and Durinian, R.A. Electroacupuncture inhibition of nocioceptive responses in the caudal trigeminal nucleus. *Biull. Eksp. Biol. Med.*, 1980, 89(1): 7–9, (in Russian).

Mu, J. Influence of adrenergic antagonist and naloxone on the antiallergenic shock effect of EAP in mice. *Am. J. Acupunc. (Abs.)*, 1986, 14:176; ex. *AETRIJ*, 1985, 10: 163–167.

Nogier, P. *De L'Auriculomedicine,* Maisonneuve, Sainte–Ruffine, France, 1981.

Oleson, T. and Kroening, R. A comparison of Chinese and Nogier auricular acupuncture points. *Am. J. Acupunc.*, Jul.–Sept. 1983, 11(3): 205–223.

Ong, L.S., Hamiadji, T., and Chong, K.L. The external ear — the electrical aspects in relation to acupuncture: a preliminary report. *Med. J. Malays*, 1980, 35(1): 53–57.

Overby, B.J. A new theory explains auricular therapy. *Deutsche Zeitschr. F. Akupunktur,* 1985, 28(5): 112–115, (in German).

Roccia, L. Current status of acupuncture and auriculotherapy. *Minerva Med.*, Dec. 1979, 15, 70(56): 3875–3887, (in Italian).

Rwshetniak, V.K. and Chuvin, B.T. Modulating effect of electric acupuncture stimulation on the biochemical activity of neurons specific and nonspecific thalamic nuclei. *Biull. Eksp. Biol. Med.*, May 1986, 101(5): 515–517, (in Russian).

Sakashita, T. *Jinshinho no Rinsho.* Taniguchi Shoten, Tokyo, 1990, (in Japanese).

Santaro, M. *L'acupuncture par L'oreille: Anatomie, Anesthesie.* Maloine, Paris, 1974, (in French).

Serizawa, K. *Clinical Acupuncture, A Practical Japanese Approach.* Japan Publications, Tokyo, 1988.

Shanghai College of Traditional Chinese Medicine. *Acupuncture, A Comprehensive Text.* Bensky, D. and O'Connor, J. (Trans. Eds.), Eastland Press, Seattle, WA, 1981.

Shapiro, R.S. and Stockard, H.E. Electroencephalographic evidence demonstrates altered brainwave patterns by acupoint stimulation. *Am. J. Acupunc.*, Jan.–Mar. 1989, 17(1).

Sin, Y.M., Chan, W.S., and Lee, E. Beneficial effects of EAP on irradiated mice. *Am. J. Acupunc.*, 1987, 15: 239–244.

Sionneau, P. and Gang, L. *The Treatment of Disease in TCM, Vol. 2. Diseases of the Eyes, Ears, Nose, and Throat*. Blue Poppy Press, Boulder, CO, 1996.

Soliman, N. and Frank, B.L. Auricular acupuncture and auricular medicine. *Phys. Med. Rehab. Clin. N. Am.*, Aug. 1999, 10(3): 547–554.

Spagnoletti, T., Liotti, M., Titino, L., Marcucci, F., Cafaro, M.R., Officioso, A., and De Luca, R. Ear-acupuncture and endocrine secretion. *Boll. Soc. Ital. Biol. Sper.*, Mar. 15, 1982, 58(5): 197–199, (in Italian).

Spoerel, W.E., Varkey, M., and Leung, C. Acupuncture in chronic pain. *Am. J. Chin. Med.*, Autumn 1976, 4(3): 267–279.

Steidl, L., Debef, J., Jandova, D., Kasparek, J., and Trneck, J. Trigeminofacial reflex. III. Effect of auriculotherapy. *Acta Univ. Palacki. Olomuc. Fac. Med.*, 1987, 117: 141–50, (in Czech).

Tanaka, T.H. The possibilities for optimizing acupuncture treatment results through synchronization with somatic state: examination of autonomic response to superficial needling during exhalation. *Am. J. Acupunc.*, 1996, 24(4): 233–239.

Tekdemir, I., Aslan, A., and Elhan, A. A clinico-anatomic study of the auricular branch of the vagus nerve and Arnold's ear cough reflex. *Surg. Radio. Anat.*, 1998, 20: 252–257.

Tekeoglu, I., Adak, B., and Ercan, M. Suppression of experimental pain by auriculopressure. *Acupunc. Med.*, 1996, 14(1): 16–18.

The People's Medical Publishing House. *Advances in Acupuncture and Acupuncture Anaesthesia.* Beijing, China, 1980.

Tsirul'nikov, E.M., Enin, L.D., and Potekhina, I.L. Focused ultrasound in research on somatic reseption. *Neirofiziologiia*, 1992, 24(5): 529–534, (in Russian).

Vashchenko, E.A., Garkavenko, V.V., and Limanskii, I.P. Modulation of the nociceptive flexor reflexes by the electrostimulation of auricular acupuncture points. *Fiziol. ZH*, Jul.–Aug. 1989, 35(4): 85–90, (in Russian).

Wang, Y.J. and Zhang, W.N. Effects of EAP on regional changes of monoamine neurotransmitters in brain of rat with carbon tetrachloride-induced liver injury. *Am. J. Acupunc. (Abs.)*, 1983, 11: 282–283; ex. JTCM, 1982, 2(Dec.): 261–265.

Xu, F., Liu, X., Liu, Z., Chen, J., and Dong, B. The role of ear electroacupuncture on arterial pressure and respiration during asphyxia in rabbits. *Zhen Ci Yan Jiu*, 1992, 17(1): 36–38, (in Chinese).

Yi, L. and Minkov, M. The external ear/embryo relationship explains the basis of ear acupuncture. *Pac. J. Orient. Med.*, 1996, 2: 20–23.

Young, M.F. and McCarthy, P.W. Effect of acupuncture stimulation of the auricular sympathetic point on evoked sudomotor response. *J. Altern. Complement. Med.*, Spring 1998, 4(1): 29–38.

Yu, J. et al. Changes in serum FSH, LH, and ovarian follicular growth during EAP for induction of ovulation. *Am. J. Acupunc. (Abs.)*, 1989, 17: 269–270, ex. CJIT and WM, 1989, 9: 199–202.

Yurino, M. et al. Clinical effect of EAP on peripheral venous circulation. *AJA* (Abs.), 1987, 15376; ex. *J. Jpn. Soc. Acupunc.*, 1986, 36: 172–177.

Zanini, F. Current role of acupuncture in analgesic therapy. *Minerva Med.*, Apr. 21, 1983, 74(17): 961–967, (in Italian).

Zhu, B., Liu, T., and Zhu, J. The alpha-dissipation characteristic of human auricular points. *Sheng Wu Yi Xue Gong Xue Za Zhi*, Mar. 2000, 17(1): 41–43, (in Chinese).

Zhu, Y., Ye, Y., and Ben, H. Effects of humoral factors in viscera-auriculopoint response in rabbits — a cross circulation experiment. *Zhen Ci Yan Jiu*, 1990, 15(4): 306–309, (in Chinese).

chapter two

The anatomical terminology of auricular medicine

Objective

- To learn the 21 anatomical zones of the ear

Introduction

Adept knowledge of ear anatomy is crucial for precise location of the ear acupuncture points. Like body acupuncture points, the location of auricular acupoints is defined in anatomical language. These definitions give the practitioner a clear roadmap as to where the points are located. This anatomical language is easy to learn and essential if one chooses to utilize the ear frequently in clinical practice. Obviously, correct ear point location is also imperative in order to achieve successful results in treatment.

Particular points are located within each ear zone, many of which are found in relation to each other. To facilitate learning these ear points, I have organized the location of 100 common ear points into 21 zones. First, the practitioner must learn the anatomical terminology for each zone of the ear. This terminology is presented below and illustrated in Figure 2.1.

Framework of the ear

21 anatomical structures

These 21 structures constitute the anatomical framework of the ear. To assist in an easy orientation to the anatomy of the ear, the structures are grouped in relation to their parts or proximity to each other.

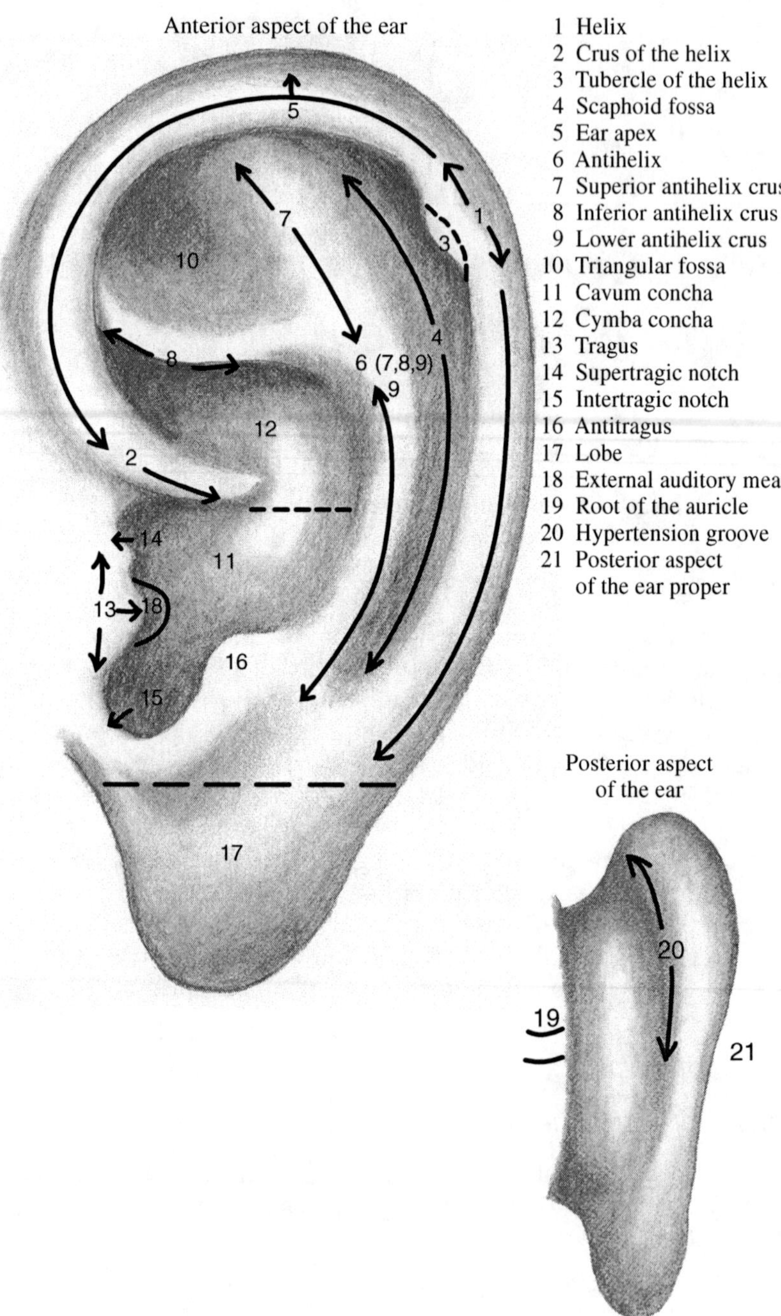

Figure 2.1 The anatomy of the ear.

Anterior aspect of the ear

Helix

1. **Helix**: The outermost portion of the auricle consisting of a rim-like structure.
2. **Crus of the helix**: The beginning of the helix. It originates in the cavum concha (see #11).
3. **Tubercle of the helix**: A small appendage on the medial border of the outer rim of the helix, approximately at the junction of the upper and middle two thirds of the helix. The tubercle of the helix is also called Darwin's tubercle. (Note: Many patients have very subtle and relatively undefined tubercles; hence, we must infer where it would be. To do this, divide the length of the ear in thirds. It is roughly at the upper third of the helix. See Figure 2.2 and Figure 2.3 for depictions of a pronounced tubercle and a tubercle that needs to be inferred.)
4. **Scaphoid fossa**: The depression between the helix and the antihelix (see #6).
5. **Ear apex**: The height of the helix. If you gently fold the ear, the ear apex is at the top where the fold occurs.

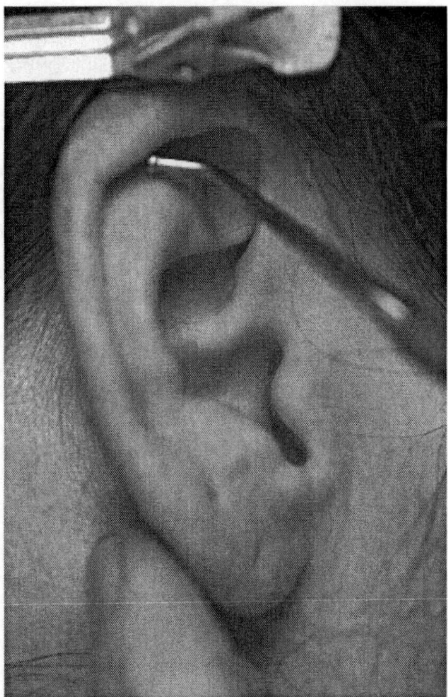

Figure 2.2 A normal tubercle of the helix.

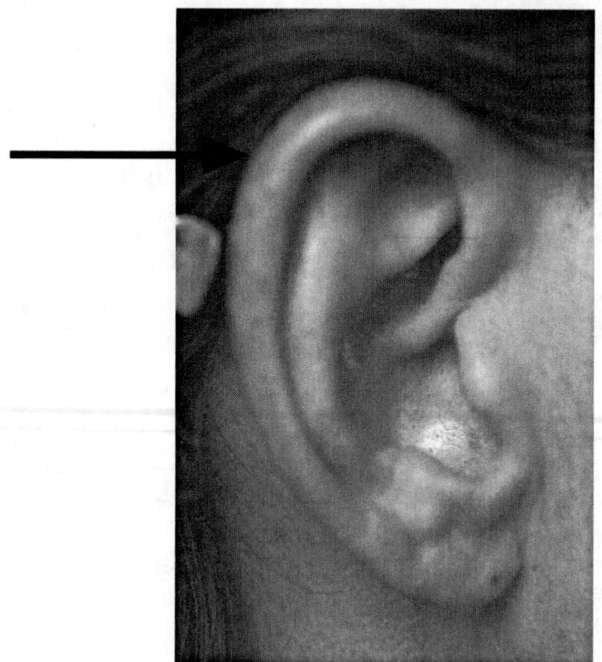

Figure 2.3 A less well-defined tubercle.

Antihelix

6. **Antihelix**: The elevated ridge-like structure medial to the helix and running parallel to it. The antihelix and the helix are separated by the scaphoid fossa. The antihelix has three parts:
7. **Superior antihelix crus:** The more lateral, superior branch of the antihelix. It bifurcates off the lower antihelix crus at the Lumbago point (see Chapter 3, #80 and Figure 3.1).
8. **Inferior antihelix crus:** The more medial, inferior branch of the antihelix. It bifurcates off of the lower antihelix crus at the Lumbago point (see Chapter 3, #80 and Figure 3.1).
9. **Lower antihelix crus:** The lower portion of the antihelix. The inferior and superior antihelix crura bifurcate off of the lower antihelix crus.
10. **Triangular fossa**: The triangular depression bordered by the superior and inferior antihelix crura.

Conchas

11. **Cavum concha**: The interior portion of the auricle that has a concave surface. It is separated from the cymba concha by the crus of the helix and lies inferior to the crus of the helix.
12. **Cymba concha**: The interior portion of the auricle that is below the inferior antihelix crus. The cymba concha lies superior to the cavum concha with the crus of the helix dividing them.

Tragus

13. **Tragus**: The small ridge-like flap connected to the lateral portion of the face. The tragus is directly anterior to the external auditory meatus.
14. **Supratragic notch**: The indentation above the tragus.
15. **Intertragic notch**: The indentation below the tragus.
16. **Antitragus**: The bump-like structure at an inferior, diagonal angle to the tragus.
17. **Lobe**: The lowest portion of the auricle. The lower border of the intertragic notch demarcates the lobe's upper border.
18. **External auditory meatus**: The canal medial to the cavum concha, behind the tragus, that conducts sound waves into the inner ear.

Posterior aspect of the ear

19. **Root of the auricle (also referred to as the Ear Root)**: The depression on the posterior aspect of the ear just above the tendinous flap that connects the auricle to the head.
20. **Hypertension groove**: A groove-like depression formed by the posterior border of the helix. The hypertension groove runs in approximately the upper third of the groove on the posterior aspect of the ear.
21. **Posterior aspect of the ear proper:** The rest fo the back of the ear.

Once these twenty-one structures, their names, and locations are committed to memory, one will have a firm foundation for locating the 100 most common ear points presented in this book. Redrawing the ear and its parts is an effective way to become familiar with the general shape of the ear and its anatomical parts.

Bibliography

Liu, S. *Auricular Diagnosis, Treatment, and Health Preservation*. Science Press, Beijing, China, 1996.

Oleson, T. *Auriculotherapy Manual: Chinese and Western Systems of Ear Acupuncture*. Health Care Alternatives, Los Angeles, 1996.

WHO. *The Report of the Working Group on Auricular Acupuncture*. World Health Organization, Lyon, France, 1990.

chapter three

The location of 100 common ear points

Objective

- To master the 100 common points of the ear in an easy fashion by organizing the points within each anatomical zone in relation to each other

Introduction

According to various authors, there are several hundred ear acupuncture points and more are being discovered through clinical research. Different authors have different preferred points. The 100 points I favor are those most commonly used in contemporary China and depicted on common ear maps, which I have modified through my own clinical experience. In the 20 years I have practiced, using the points and charts that comprise this book, I have never needed to consult another ear chart to find new points in order to address a diagnosis. The simple Chinese ear map has always met my needs of providing accurate, efficient, and effective healthcare for my patients.

As a microsystem, almost all anatomical sites, visceral organs, and system parts are represented on the ear. Points are conventionally named according to the organ, body part, or physiological role that they play in the body. If a point is not found on the ear map, you can always infer where that point location might be. For instance, if the patient has a charley horse in his or her calf and there is no calf point in the ear map system, one can predict that the calf point would be midway between the ankle point and the knee point, just as the calf actually is midway between the knee and the ankle on the leg.

Figure 3.1 and Figure 3.2 depict the left ear and right ear (respectively) of a patient. As individuals, patients have variations in auricular size and shape, but the ear parts or zones are present on all ears unless there is a

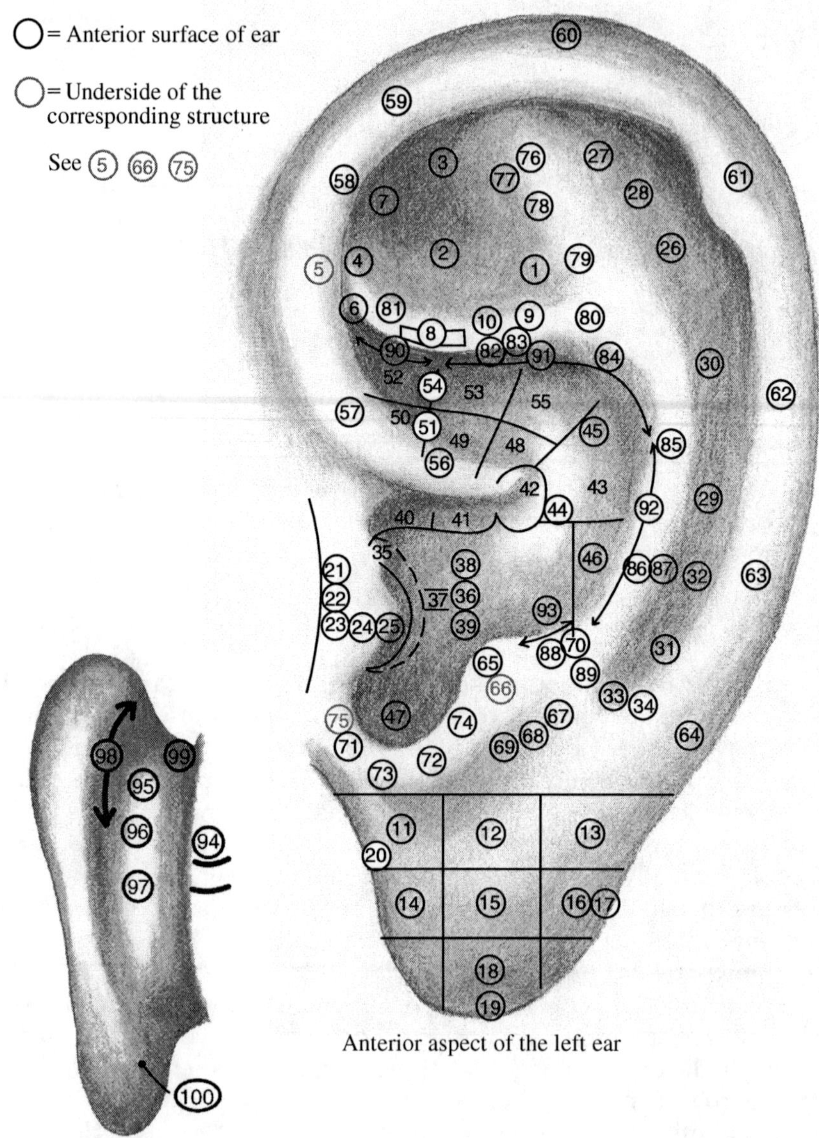

Figure 3.1 Contemporary Chinese ear map (left ear).

congenital or pathological abnormality. Therefore, the points can all be found through a familiarity with the 21 anatomical ear zones. The instructions on how to locate points are found below. Some points are small in size, while others are larger; these are described as areas.

For clinician convenience, three tables are provided for the reader. In Table 3.1, the 100 points are first distributed according to anatomical zone.

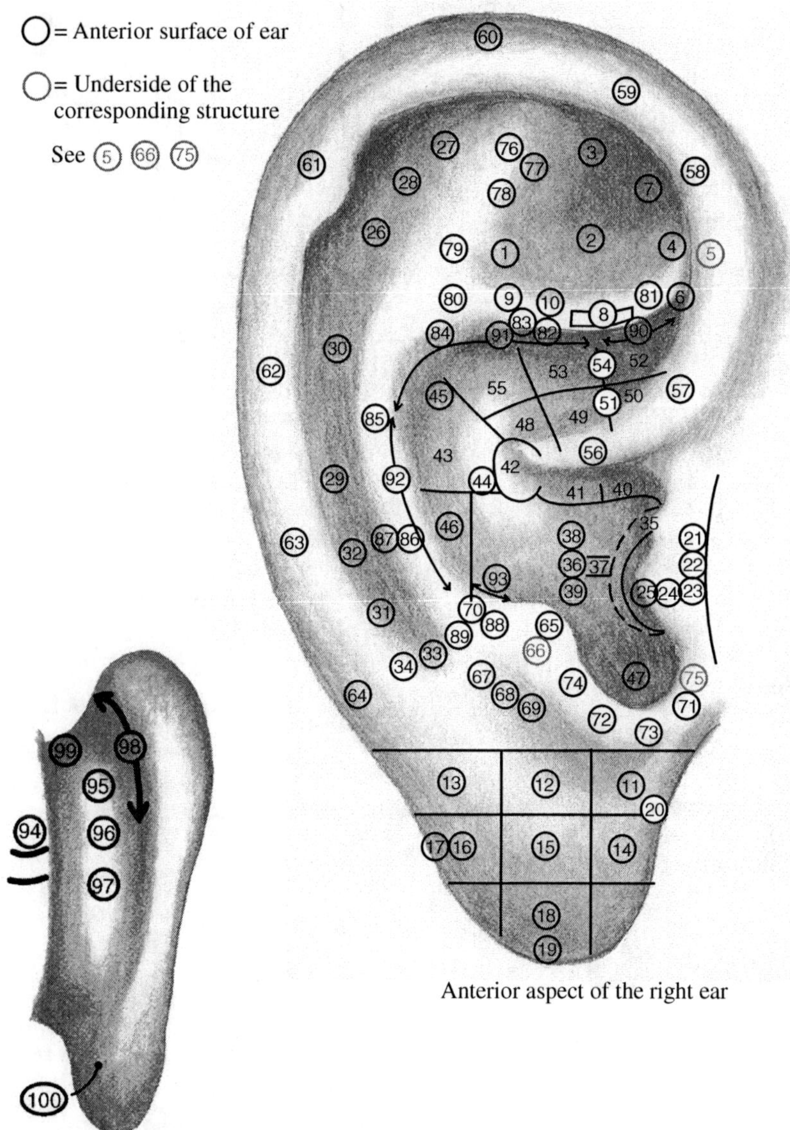

Figure 3.2 Ear points of the right ear.

Next, they are assigned numbers. These numbers are the same numbers assigned to each point in Figure 3.1 and Figure 3.2. For instance, by looking at this chart, the reader can see all of the points that are found in the cavum concha, such as Point 36, the Heart.

Table 3.2 is a handy alphabetical index of ear acupuncture point names. If looking for the Heart point, for example, simply look it up alphabetically

Table 3.1 Ear Point Location by Number

Points of the Triangular Fossa (G)	
1	*Shenmen*
2	Stop Wheezing
3	Hypertension
4	Sympathetic 1
5	Sympathetic 2
6	Sympathetic 3
7	Uterus/Prostate
8	Constipation
9	Hepatitis
10	Hip Joint
Points of the Lobe (P)	
11	Upper Teeth
12	Tongue
13	Jaw
14	Lower Teeth
15	Eye
16	Inner Ear
17	Helix 5
18	Tonsil
19	Helix 6
20	Insomnia
Points of the Tragus (J)	
21	Thirst
22	External Nose
23	Hunger
24	Internal Nose
25	Adrenal
Points of the Scaphoid Fossa (O)	
26	Wrist
27	Finger
28	Allergy
29	Shoulder
30	Elbow
31	Clavicle
32	Shoulder Joint
33	Thyroid
34	Nephritis
Points of the Cavum Concha (H)	
35	Mouth
36	Heart
37	Trachea
38	Upper Lung
39	Lower Lung
40	Esophagus
41	Cardiac Sphincter
42	Stomach
43	Liver
44	Hepatitis
45	Relax Muscle
46	Spleen
47	*Sanjiao*
Points of the Cymba Concha (I)	
48	Duodenum
49	Small Intestine
50	Large Intestine
51	Appendix
52	Bladder
53	Kidney
54	Ureters
55	Pancreas/Gallbladder
Points of the Helix and Crus of Helix (A & B)	
56	Diaphragm
57	Lower Portion of the Rectum
58	Hemorrhoids
59	Common Cold
60	Ear Apex
61	Helix 1
62	Helix 2
63	Helix 3
64	Helix 4
Points of the Antitragus and Intertragic Notch (L & M)	
65	*Dingchuan*
66	Brain
67	Occiput
68	Temple
69	Forehead
70	Brainstem
71	Eye 1
72	Eye 2
73	Raise Blood Pressure
74	Ovaries/Testes
75	Endocrine
Points of the Superior Antihelix Crus (D)	
76	Toe
77	Heel
78	Ankle
79	Knee
80	Lumbago

Table 3.1 (continued) Ear Point Location by Number

Points of the Inferior Antihelix Crus (E)	
81	Sciatic Nerve
82	Ischium
83	Buttocks
Points of the Lower Antihelix Crus (F)	
84	Abdomen
85	Chest
86–87	Mammary Glands
88	Neck
89	Throat and Teeth
90	Sacral Vertebrae
91	Lumbar Vertebrae
92	Thoracic Vertebrae
93	Cervical Vertebrae
Points on the Back of the Ear (U)	
94	Vagus Root
95	Upper Back
96	Middle Back
97	Lower Back
98	Lower Blood Pressure Groove
99	Superior Root of Ear
100	Spinal Cord 1

Table 3.2 Alphabetical Cross-Reference of Ear Points by Point Name

Anatomical Ear Zone Location:		
A. Helix	Abdomen	F 84
B. Crus of Helix	Adrenal	J 25
C. Antihelix	Allergy	O 28
D. Superior Antihelix Crus	Ankle	D 78
E. Inferior Antihelix Crus	Appendix	I 51
F. Lower Antihelix Crus	Bladder	I 52
G. Triangular Fossa	Brain	M 56
H. Cavum Concha	Brainstem	M 70
I. Cymba Concha	Buttocks	D 83
J. Tragus	Cardiac Sphincter	H 41
K. Supratragic Notch	Cervical Vertebrae	F 94
L. Intertragic Notch	Chest	F 85
M. Antitragus	Clavicle	O 31
N. Tubercle of the Helix	Common Cold	A 59
O. Scaphoid Fossa	Constipation	G 8
P. Lobe	Diaphragm	B 56
Q. Ear Apex	*Dingchuan*	M 65
R. External Auditory Meatus	Duodenum	I 48
S. Root of the Auricle	Ear Apex	A 60

(*continued*)

Table 3.2 (continued) Alphabetical Cross-Reference of Ear Points by Point

T. Hypertension Groove	Elbow	O 30
	Endocrine	M 75
	Esophagus	H 40
	External Nose	J 22
	Eye	P 15
	Eye I	M 71
	Eye II	M 72
	Finger	O 27
	Forehead	M 69
	Heart	H 36
	Heel	D 77
	Helix 1	A 61
	Helix 2	A 62
	Helix 3	A 63
	Helix 4	A 64
	Helix 5	P 17
	Helix 6	P 19
	Hemorrhoids	A 58
	Hepatitis	H 44/G 9
	Hip Joint	G 10
	Hunger	J 23
	Hypertension	G 3
	Inner Ear	P 16
	Insomnia	P 20
	Internal Nose	J 24
	Ischium	D 82
	Jaw	P 13
	Kidney	I 53
	Knee	D 79
	Large Intestine	I 50
	Liver	H 43
	Lower Back	S 97
	Lower Blood Pressure Groove	S 98
	Lower Lung	H 39
	Lower Portion of Rectum	B 57
	Lower Teeth	P 14
	Lumbago	D 80
	Lumbar Vertebrae	F 91
	Mammary Glands	F 86,87
	Middle Back	S 96
	Mouth	H 35
	Neck	F 88
	Nephritis	O 34
	Occiput	M 67
	Ovaries/Testes	M 74
	Pancreas/Gallbladder	I 55
	Raise Blood Pressure	M 73
	Relax Muscle	H 45

Table 3.2 (continued) Alphabetical Cross-Reference of Ear Points by Point

Point	Location
Sacral Vertebrae	F 90
Sanjiao	H 47
Sciatic Nerve	D 81
Shenmen	G 1
Shoulder	O 29
Shoulder Joint	O 32
Small Intestine	I 49
Spinal Cord I	U 100
Spleen	H 46
Stomach	H 42
Stop Wheezing	G 2
Superior Root of Ear	U 99
Sympathetic (1, 2, 3)	G 4,5,6
Temple	M 68
Thirst	J 21
Thoracic Vertebrae	F 93
Throat and Teeth	F 89
Thyroid	O 33
Toe	D 76
Tongue	P 12
Tonsil	P 18
Trachea	H 37
Upper Back	U 95
Upper Lung	H 38
Upper Teeth	P 11
Ureters	I 54
Uterus/Prostate	G 7
Vagus Root	U 94
Wrist	O 26

and you can see that it is number 36; it is also found in the cavum concha, which is designated by the prefix H. The H references the cavum concha in the Anatomical Ear Zone Location list.

Finally, Table 3.3 lists the points within areas of the ear by letter and number. For instance, if you were looking at the ear map and you saw a point on the helix and its number was 58, you could combine that information and use this chart to see that A58 is the Hemorrhoids point.

As a general orientation to the ear, Henry Liu maintains that "the external ear is like a dynamic hologram."[1] That hologram was described by Paul Nogier, who contended that there is a resemblance between the distribution of auricular points and the fetus in an inverted position. Thus, the head and its structures are located on the lobe; the organs are found in the conchas; and the toes, heels, and ankles (points of the lower limbs) are in the upper part of the ear; etc. This conceptualization provides us with a basic orientation to the positioning of ear points.

While there is a high degree of correspondence between the point locations of both systems advanced by the Chinese and by Nogier, there are

Table 3.3 Location Reference by Areas of the Ear

Anatomical Ear Zone Location:		
A. Helix	Hemorrhoids	A 58
B. Crus of Helix	Common Cold	A 59
C. Antihelix	Ear Apex	A 60
D. Superior Antihelix Crus	Helix 1	A 61
E. Inferior Antihelix Crus	Helix 2	A 62
F. Lower Antihelix Crus	Helix 3	A 63
G. Triangular Fossa	Helix 4	A 64
H. Cavum Concha	Diaphragm	B 56
I. Cymba Concha	Lower Portion of Rectum	B 77
J. Tragus	Toe	D 76
K. Supratragic Notch	Heel	D 77
L. Intertragic Notch	Ankle	D 78
M. Antitragus	Knee	D 79
N. Tubercle of the Helix	Lumbago	D 80
O. Scaphoid Fossa	Sciatic Nerve	D 81
P. Lobe	Ischium	D 82
Q. Ear Apex	Buttocks	D 83
R. External Auditory Meatus	Abdomen	F 84
S. Root of the Auricle	Chest	F 85
T. Hypertension Groove	Mammary Glands	F 86,87
U. Posterior Aspect of Ear	Neck	F 88
Proper	Throat and Teeth	F 89
	Sacral Vertebrae	F 90
	Lumbar Vertebrae	F 91
	Thoracic Vertebrae	F 93
	Cervical Vertebrae	F 94
	Shenmen	G 1
	Stop Wheezing	G 2
	Hypertension	G 3
	Sympathetic (1, 2, 3)	G 4,5,6
	Uterus/Prostate	G 7
	Constipation	G 8
	Hip Joint	G 9
	Mouth	H 35
	Heart	H 36
	Trachea	H 37
	Upper Lung	H 38
	Lower Lung	H 39
	Esophagus	H 40
	Cardiac Sphincter	H 41
	Stomach	H 42
	Liver	H 43
	Hepatitis	H 44/G 10
	Relax Muscle	H 45
	Spleen	H 46
	Sanjiao	H 47

Table 3.3 (continued) Location Reference by Areas of the Ear

	Duodenum	I 48
	Small Intestine	I 49
	Large Intestine	I 50
	Appendix	I 51
	Bladder	I 52
	Kidney	I 53
	Ureters	I 54
	Pancreas/Gallbladder	I 55
	Thirst	J 21
	External Nose	J 22
	Hunger	J 23
	Internal Nose	J 24
	Adrenal	J 25
	Brain	M 56
	Dingchuan	M 65
	Occiput	M 67
	Temple	M 68
	Forehead	M 69
	Brainstem	M 70
	Eye I	M 71
	Eye II	M 72
	Raise Blood Pressure	M 73
	Ovaries/Testes	M 74
	Endocrine	M 75
	Wrist	O 26
	Finger	O 27
	Allergy	O 28
	Shoulder	O 29
	Elbow	O 30
	Clavicle	O 31
	Shoulder Joint	O 32
	Thyroid	O 33
	Nephritis	O 34
	Upper Teeth	P 11
	Tongue	P 12
	Jaw	P 13
	Lower Teeth	P 14
	Eye	P 15
	Inner Ear	P 16
	Helix 5	P 17
	Tonsil	P 18
	Helix 6	P 19
	Insomnia	P 20
	Vagus Root	U 94
	Upper Back	U 95
	Middle Back	U 96
	Lower Back	U 97

(*continued*)

Table 3.3 (continued) Location Reference by Areas of the Ear

	Lower Blood Pressure Groove	U 98
	Superior Root of Ear	U 99
	Spinal Cord I	U 100

some differences. Nogier's system tends to emphasize the organization of the points more by the nervous system than by the meridian system.[2] He locates some of the points in different places from the Chinese map, such as the Heart, Kidney, Spleen, and Adrenal points. His system can be consulted if the reader chooses. However, there are more similarities than differences. As a reminder, please note that the purpose of this book is not to illustrate or reconcile the differences between the Chinese vs. Nogier systems. My strength and specialty is the particular Chinese ear map and, hopefully, the ability to make ear acupuncture medicine uncomplicated for the practitioner.

With the 100 most common ear points locations, it is best to begin with *Shenmen* because it the most important point in the ear. Since it is located in the triangular fossa, I start by numbering the points within the triangular fossa. In addition to the point location descriptions, clinical tips for locating some of these points are presented where relevant.

10 points of the triangular fossa (G): points that relate to nervous and hormonal regulation and the pelvic organs

Location tip

Locating the borders of the triangular fossa — When one is first learning auricular point location, it is sometimes difficult to perceive the borders of the triangular fossa, especially its upper border. If you do not know the borders of the triangular fossa you cannot locate the points correctly within it. First, remember that the triangular fossa is a depression. Relatively speaking, it is usually a slightly darker hue than the tissue of the superior and inferior antihelix cruras. During pregnancy and menstruation, the triangular fossa is oftentimes a bright red. If the patient has painful periods, it tends to be on the dark side. One of my students had a permanent blue triangular fossa on one side of one ear. When I inquired about it, she said that she was deprived of oxygen at the time of her birth. (Interestingly, the Stop Wheezing point pertaining to respiration is in the center of the triangular fossa).

A simple tip that can help with demarcating the triangular fossa's upper border is to gently press the helix of the ear inward (medially). When you do this, the superior antihelix crus becomes more visible and elevated, thus making the triangular fossa's upper border clearly demarcated (Figure 3.3).

1. ***Shenmen***: Located in the triangular fossa along the lateral border, superior to the junction of its inferior and superior borders. Place the ear probe in this juncture and then slide superiorly to the intersection. The probe will fall into a small depression; that is the point.

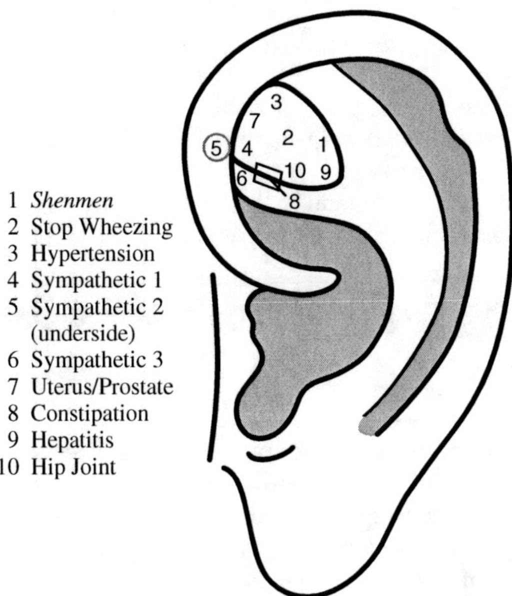

Figure 3.3 Points of the triangular fossa (G).

2. **Stop Wheezing**: Located in the deepest point in the center of the triangular fossa. Place the probe roughly in this vicinity. Search by feel with the probe for the depression which is where the point is located.
3. **Hypertension**: Located in the laterosuperior corner of the triangular fossa.

Notes: There are three standard locations of the Sympathetic point. One of them is actually in the triangular fossa, another is on the posterior border of the helix, and the third is below the triangular fossa. However, I have included the latter two here because they are alternative locations for what I am designating as Sympathetic 1. I have labeled them as follows:

4. **Sympathetic 1**: Located in the medioinferior corner of the triangular fossa.
5. **Sympathetic 2**: Located on the posterior border of the helix, midway between the level of Sympathetic 1 and Sympathetic 3. This is the first of three points on my map that are located on the posterior border of an ear structure.
6. **Sympathetic 3**: Located on the inferior antihelix crus, below Sympathetic 1.
7. **Uterus/Prostate (seminal vesicle)**: Located midway between Sympathetic 1 and the Hypertension point.

8. **Constipation**: Located on the inferior border of the triangular fossa. This point is an area equivalent to a rectangular shape. Part of it is along the inferior border of the triangular fossa and part is along the upper portion of the inferior antihelix crus.
9. **Hepatitis**: Located at the junction of the inferior and superior borders of the triangular fossa.
10. **Hip Joint**: Located medial to the Hepatitis point, on the lower border of the triangular fossa.

10 points of the lobe (P): points of the head and face

Location tip

Dividing the lobe into sectors — in order to find the points located on the lobe, the upper border of the lobe must be established. Mentally, or using the ear probe as a straight edge, draw a horizontal line across the lobe at the level of the lower border of the intertragic notch, which has a lip-like cartilaginous shape to it. It is from there that the horizontal line is drawn and the upper border of the lobe is created.

After locating the upper border of the lobe (see Figure 3.4), divide the lobe into equal thirds vertically and then equal thirds horizontally. This division can be done visually or using an ear probe as a straight edge. Nine sectors are then formed on the lobe (see Figure 3.5). These sectors are universally assigned numbers 1 through 9 as you read from left to right and top to bottom. The points are located in relation to these sectors. Most of these points are defined as, *"In the center of the _th sector."* For example, the Eye point is located in the center of the 5th sector.

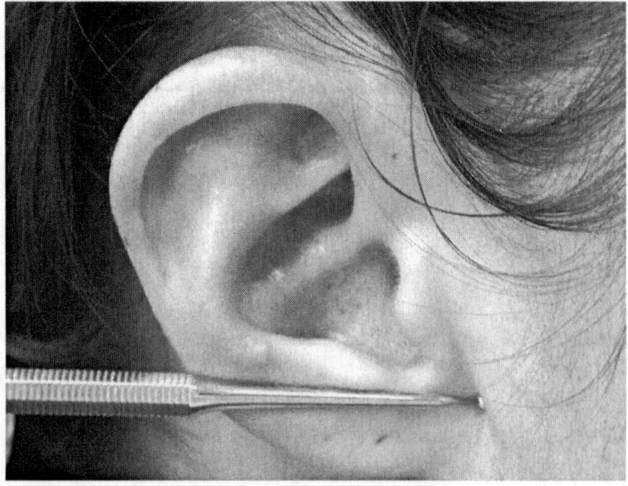

Figure 3.4 How to locate the upper margin of the lobe.

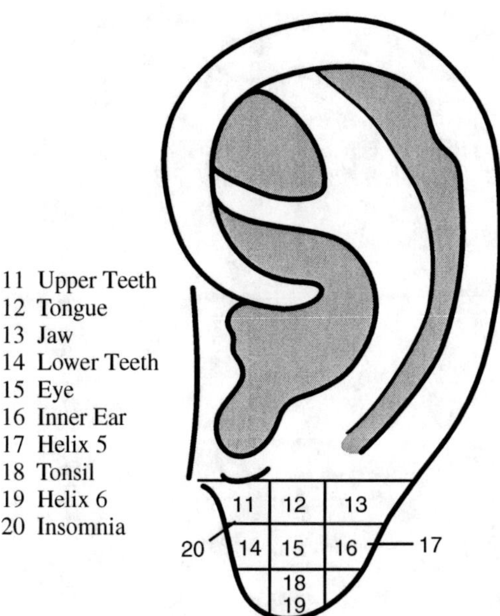

Figure 3.5 Points of the lobe (P).

11. **Upper Teeth**: Located slightly below the center of Sector 1.
12. **Tongue**: Located in the center of Sector 2.
13. **Jaw**: Located in the center of Sector 3.
14. **Lower Teeth**: Located in the center of Sector 4.
15. **Eye**: Located in the center of Sector 5.
16. **Inner Ear**: Located in the center of Sector 6.
17. **Helix 5**: Located on the lateral border of Sector 6.
18. **Tonsil**: Located in the center of Sector 8.
19. **Helix 6:** Located on the lower margin of Sector 8.
20. **Insomnia**: Located slightly medial to the teeth points (#11 and #14), on the horizontal line dividing the Upper Teeth (#11) and Lower Teeth points (#14).

5 points of the tragus (J): points that pertain to hormonal regulation

Location tip

The tragus may be made up of one or two lobes. If there are two, they are created by an indentation between the lobes. Many patients have a small tragus, and it may be difficult to see the indentation. Sometimes the patient only has one lobe; hence, the practitioner must infer where an indentation would occur. Figure 3.6 shows a well-defined tragus, and Figure 3.7 shows one that is less defined, and how to visualize where an indentation would fall.

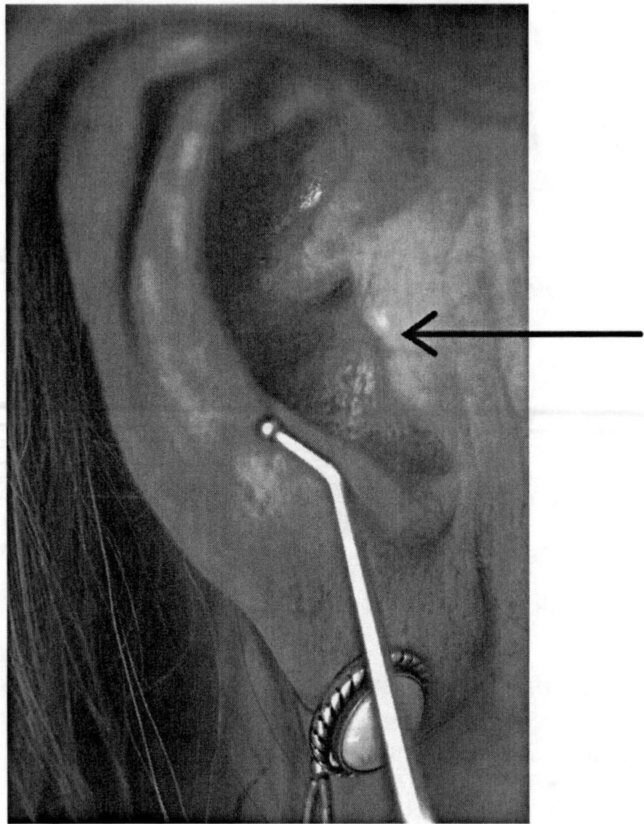

Figure 3.6 The arrow denotes a well-defined tragus. The probe is on the groove of the neck point.

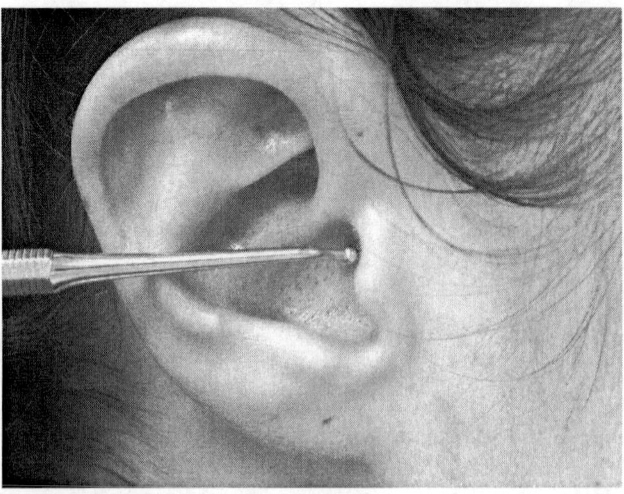

Figure 3.7 A tragus that is less defined and a visualized indentation.

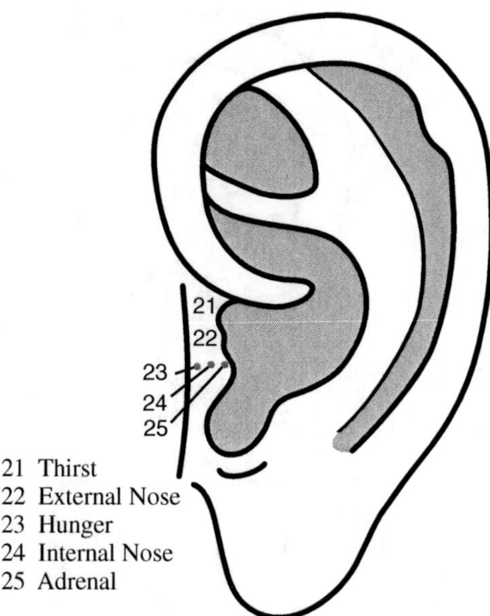

Figure 3.8 Points of the tragus (J).

> ***Note:*** Some texts do not align points 21 to 23. However, the Chinese doctors with whom I studied in Beijing used these locations as I do (Figure 3.8).

21. **Thirst**: Located in the center of the superior portion of the tragus.
22. **External Nose**: Located midway between the Thirst and Hunger points, in the center of the tragus.
23. **Hunger**: Located on the lower lobe of the tragus, directly below the External Nose point.
24. **Internal Nose**: Located midway between the Hunger and Adrenal points on the lower portion of the tragus.
25. **Adrenal**: Located on the lower portion of the tragus close to its lateral border.

9 points of the scaphoid fossa (O): points of the upper limb

Location tip

The definition of these points begins with *"Located in the scapha …."* Most of these points are located in relation to each other, and so it is necessary to know how to define each point (Figure 3.9).

26. **Wrist**: Located in the scapha, opposite the tubercle of the helix.
27. **Finger**: Located in the scapha in its uppermost portion. The points are an area vs. a single point. I picture this area like the length of extended fingers.

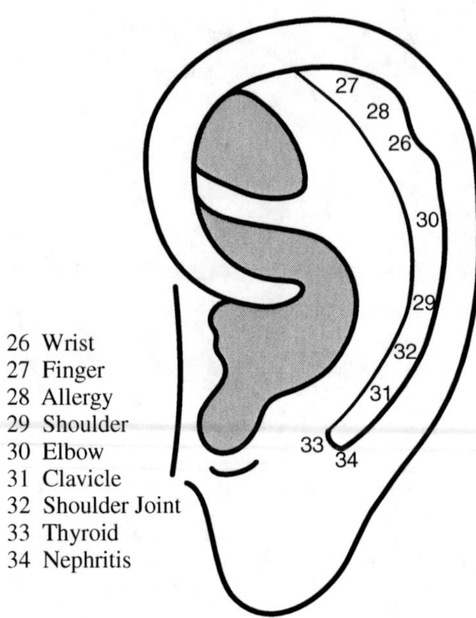

Figure 3.9 Points of the scaphoid fossa (O).

28. **Allergy**: Located in the scapha, midway between the Wrist and Finger points.
29. **Shoulder**: Located in the scapha, level with the crus of the helix. Some texts place this point at the level of the supratragic notch.
30. **Elbow**: Located in the scapha, midway between the Wrist and the Shoulder points.
31. **Clavicle**: Located in the scapha, level with the height of the antitragus. Some sources place the Clavicle point as level with the notch above the antitragus.
32. **Shoulder Joint**: Located in the scapha, midway between the Shoulder and Clavicle points.
33. **Thyroid**: Located on the medial border of the scapha, parallel but slightly inferior to the Throat and Teeth point (see point F 89).
34. **Nephritis**: Located below the Clavicle point, at the end of the lateral border of the scapha.

13 points of the cavum concha (H): organs of the thoracic region

35. **Mouth**: This area curves like a smile to parallel the lateral border of the external auditory meatus.
36. **Heart**: Located at the deepest point of the cavum concha, at the level of the center of the Mouth point. Eyeball this area, put the

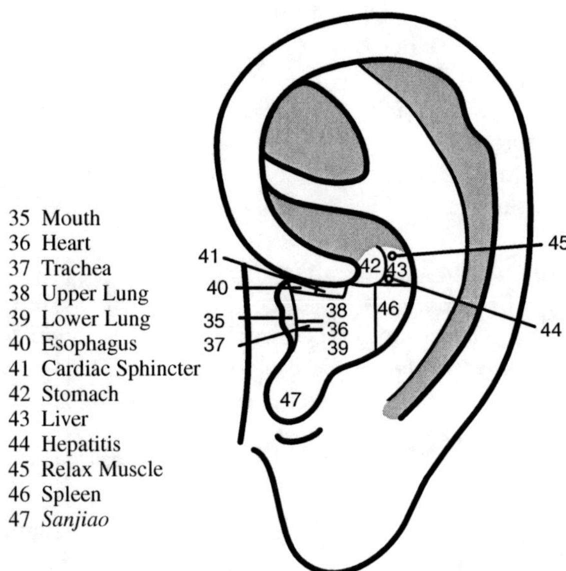

Figure 3.10 Points of the cavum concha (H).

probe in the cavum concha, and then search with the probe for the deepest point.

37. **Trachea**: A narrow horizontal area that starts at the center of the Mouth point and extends to the Heart point.
38. **Upper Lung**: Located in the depression above the Heart point. Put the ear probe in the Heart point, and then slide slightly above it until the probe falls into a depression. The Upper Lung point is in the depression.
39. **Lower Lung**: Located in the depression below the Heart point. Put the probe on the Heart point, and then slide slightly below it until the probe falls into a depression. The Lower Lung point is in the depression.
40. **Esophagus:** Take the length of the distance from the upper curvature of the Mouth point to the lateral end of the lower border of the crus of the helix. Divide this distance in half. The most medial half is the Esophagus area.
41. **Cardiac Sphincter**: See the location of point 40. The half that is lateral to the Esophagus point is the Cardiac sphincter area.
42. **Stomach**: The Stomach point is a round area that begins at the end of the crus of the helix and extends halfway across the distance formed by the end of the crus and the medial border of the lower antihelix crus. Because pathology in the Stomach area can change the shape of the Stomach point (discussed in Chapter 7), we need to know exactly where it ends in order to precisely locate the point.The best way to locate the Stomach point is as follows. Place

the ear probe on the Diaphragm point (point B 56), and then slide off the crus of the helix. The probe will fall into a little notch that can be felt with the probe. That notch is the beginning of the Stomach area. The Stomach area, in the shape of a semicircle, extends halfway across the distance from this notch to the medial border of the lower antihelix crus.

43. **Liver**: The Liver comprises the second half of the distance from the Stomach point to the medial border of the lower antihelix crus. The area is triangular in shape. Its superior border is formed by a 45-degree angle from the upper border of the Stomach point to the medial border of the lower antihelix crus. The Liver's lower border is level with the lower border of the crus of the helix.
44. **Hepatitis**: This point is an area found within the Liver area, close to the lateral curvature of the Stomach.
45. **Relax Muscle**: This point is also within the Liver area. It lies in a roughly circular area below the superior border of the Liver area.
46. **Spleen**: This point is a large area. First locate the midpoint of the lower border of the Liver. Now extend a line vertically downward to where the line intersects with the curvature superior to the antitragus. The area lateral to the line is the Spleen area.
47. ***Sanjiao* (Triple Warmer)**: This point is located in the deepest area of the cavum concha, at the level of the intertragic notch. To locate this point, "look" through the intertragic notch as if it were a small window. Then place the ear probe within it, and feel for the deepest depression. That is the *Sanjiao* point.

8 points of the cymba concha (I): the abdominal organ points

Location tip

The points of the cymba concha are located in relation to each other, as are the points of the cavum concha and scaphoid fossa. Each point is located in a sector. Divide the length of the cymba concha horizontally in half following the natural curvature of the cymba concha. Then diagonally divide the cymba concha equally into thirds as illustrated in Figure 3.11. This produces six sectors in the cymba concha. They are named as sectors #1, #2, and #3, going from lateral to medial in the lower half of the cymba concha. Sectors #4, #5, and #6 are numbered from medial to lateral in the upper half of the cymba concha.

48. **Duodenum**: Located in the 1st sector.
49. **Small Intestine**: Located in the 2nd sector.
50. **Large Intestine**: Located in the 3rd sector.
51. **Appendix**: Located at the junction of the 2nd and 3rd sectors (between the Small Intestine and the Large Intestine points).

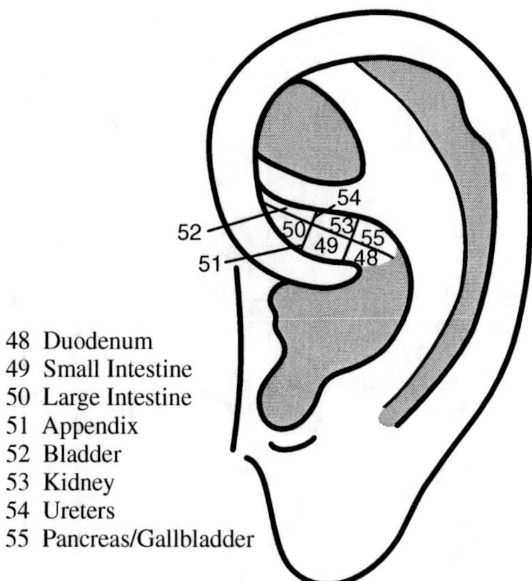

Figure 3.11 Points of the cymba concha (I).

52. **Bladder**: Located in the 4th sector directly above the Large Intestine point.
53. **Kidney**: Located in the 5th sector directly above the Small Intestine point.
54. **Ureters**: Located at the junction of the 4th and 5th sectors (between the Kidney and Bladder points).
55. **Pancreas/Gallbladder**: Located in the 6th sector directly above the Duodenum point. The Chinese say the Gallbladder point is located in the right ear and the Pancreas point in the left ear. Hans Ulrich Hecker makes a further discrimination by maintaining that "the head of the pancreas is also projected on the right ear, while the body and the tail are projected on the left."[3] I do not make these distinctions, but rather equally treat both the pancreas and the gallbladder through each ear.

9 points of the helix (A) and the crus of the helix (B): assorted points and points of the lower portion of the body

56. **Diaphragm**: Located near the lateral edge of the crus of the helix.
57. **Lower Portion of the Rectum**: Located on the helix, roughly parallel to the Large Intestine point.
58. **Hemorrhoids**: Located on the border of the helix, parallel to the Uterus/Prostate point(#7).
59. **Common Cold**: Located on the border of the helix, parallel to the Hypertension point.

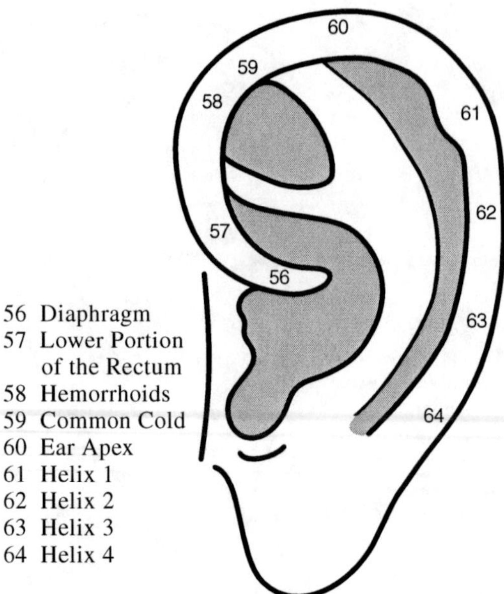

Figure 3.12 Points of the helix and crus of the helix (A and B).

60. **Ear Apex**: The point is at the apex of the helix of the ear. The apex is found by gently folding the helix.

61., 62., 63., 64. **Helixes 1 to 4**: These points are found by dividing the helix horizontally into six equal parts. (Helixes 5 and 6 have already been numbered as point #17 and point #19, respectively.) The first point is on the helix, parallel to the tubercle of the helix and the sixth point is found in Sector 8 of the lobe. All of the others are found in between those divisions at equal intervals.

11 points of the antitragus (M) and intertragic notch area (L): points of the head and brain regions

65. ***Dingchuan:*** Located at the height of the antitragus (not on the anterior surface, but exactly on the top of the antitragus).

66. **Brain (also known as Subcortex)**: Located on the posterior wall of the antitragus. Some sources make a distinction between the Brain and the Subcortex; however, I do not. In the former case, they put the Subcortex on the posterior wall of the antitragus, and the Brain midway between the Brainstem point (point #70) and *Dingchuan*. This is the second point on my map that is located on the posterior aspect of an ear part.

67., 68., 69. **Occiput, Temple, and Forehead**: These three points are found inferior to the antitragus. They run parallel to it on a curve. The most lateral one is Occiput, Temple is in the middle, and Forehead is the most medial.

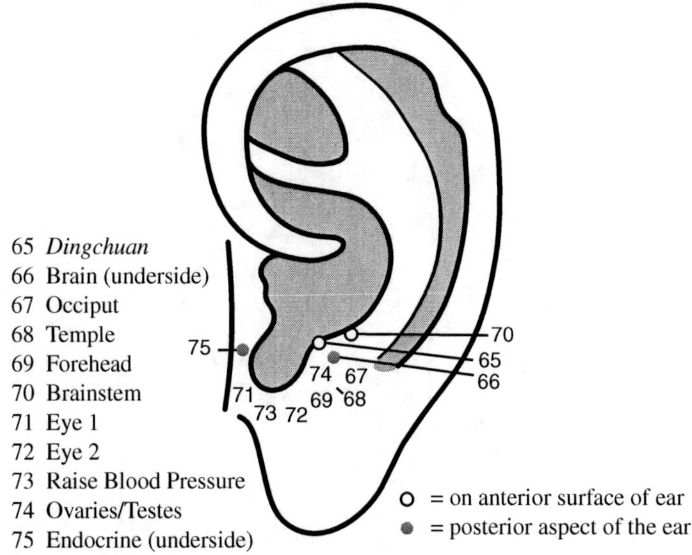

Figure 3.13 Points of the antitragus and intertragic notches (L and M).

70. **Brainstem**: This point is located just above the antitragus area, at the intersection of the medial border of the Spleen point with the curvature above the antitragus.
71. **Eye 1**: Located on the medial side of the intertragic notch.
72. **Eye 2**: Located on the lateral side of the intertragic notch.
73. **Raise Blood Pressure**: This point is located below the intertragic notch between Eye 1 and Eye 2.
74. **Ovaries/Testes**: These points are located slightly superior to Eye 2. Some sources locate the Ovary point on the lower medial interior portion of the antitragus.
75. **Endocrine**: This point is located on the medial side of the intertragic notch superior to Eye 1, on the posterior wall of the medial border of the intertragic notch. This is the third and final point on my map that is not on the anterior surface of the ear.

Points of the antihelix (C)

5 points of the superior antihelix crus (D): points of the lower limb

Location tip

Toe, heel, ankle — these three points are most easily located in relation to each other. In looking at the left ear of a person, these points form an inverted L.

76. **Toe**: The most lateral point, found where the inverted L begins.
77. **Heel**: Located at the junction of the two strokes that form the L.

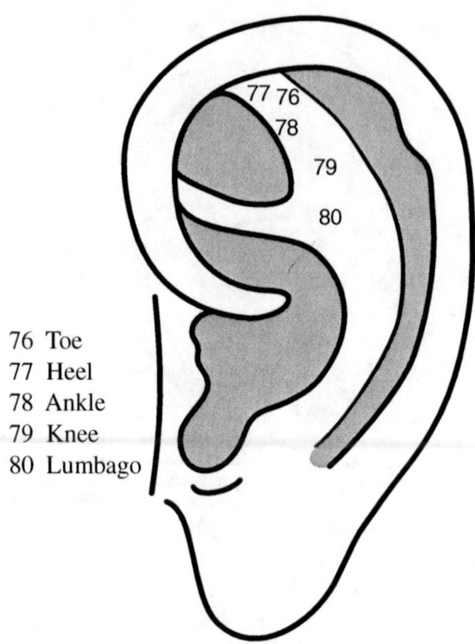

Figure 3.14 Points of the superior antihelix crus (D).

78. **Ankle**: Located inferior to the Heel point where the inverted L ends.
79. **Knee**: This is an area superior to where the superior antihelix crus intersects with the inferior antihelix crus.
80. **Lumbago**: This point is found exactly at the intersection of the superior and inferior antihelix crura.

3 points of the inferior antihelix crus (E): points of the lower limb

81. **Sciatic Nerve**: Located at the medial end of the inferior antihelix crus.
82. **Ischium**: Located just below the triangular fossa in the inferior antihelix crus, slightly medial to the Buttocks point.
83. **Buttocks**: Located just below the triangular fossa in the inferior antihelix crus, slightly lateral to the Ischium point.

10 points of the lower antihelix crus (F): thoracic cavity

84. **Abdomen**: This is an area on the lower antihelix crus roughly parallel to the Liver and Pancreas/Gallbladder points.
85. **Chest**: This is an area in the lower antihelix crus parallel to the Stomach point. Some sources describe the Chest point as level with the supratragic notch.

86., 87. **Mammary Points**: Located below the Chest area, parallel to the center of the Spleen point. There are two mammary points; they are positioned side by side.

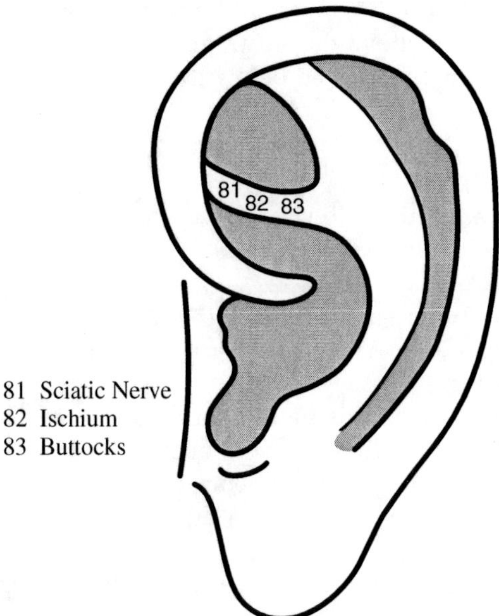

Figure 3.15 Points of the inferior antihelix crus (E).

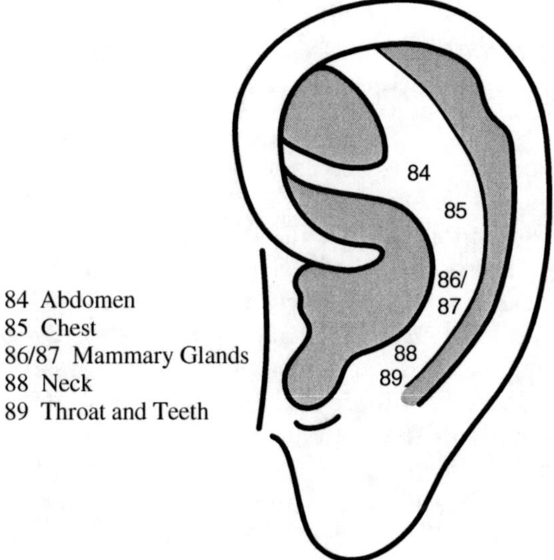

Figure 3.16 Points of the lower antihelix crus (F).

88. **Neck**: Located on the lower antihelix crus, parallel to the curvature of the antihelix, above the antitragus.
89. **Throat and Teeth**: Located below the Neck point, slightly above the Occiput point.

Location tip

The spinal points are found along the spine of the ear (or the medial edge of the inferior and lower antihelix crura).

90. **Sacral Vertebrae**: This is an area that extends from the most medial portion of the inferior antihelix crus about parallel to the end of the Bladder point.
91. **Lumbar Vertebrae**: This vertebral segment extends from the end of the Sacral vertebrae to roughly parallel to the middle of the Liver area.
92. **Thoracic Vertebrae**: This segment goes from the end of the Lumbar vertebrae to just above the curvature of the lower antihelix crus.
93. **Cervical Vertebrae**: This portion extends from the end of the Thoracic vertebrae to the end of the curvature of the lower antihelix crus.

Location Tip

Some sources recommend locating the vertebral points in the following way. Draw a line from the Lower Portion of the Rectum point (#57) to where it intersects with the antihelix. The area superior to the line is the lumbosacral area. Draw a line from the Shoulder point to where it intersects with the antihelix crus. The area superior to it is the Thoracic area and the area beneath it is the Cervical area.

7 points on the back of the ear (U): vagus nerve, blood pressure, back pain, and brain function

94. **Vagus**: Located in the depression just above the ear root (where the ear attaches to the head, above the tendon). To locate the point, gently pull the ear laterally. This will isolate the tendon to assist in locating the point. The point is in the depression above the tendon.

95., 96., 97. **Upper Back, Middle Back, and Lower Back**: These three points are located along the spiny middle portion of the back of the ear. According to *Chinese Acupuncture and Moxibustion,* the Upper Back point is on top, the Middle Back point is in the middle, and the Lower Back point is on the bottom. However, according to Bensky and O'Connor in *Acupuncture, A Comprehensive Text,* the Lower Back is on the top, the Middle Back is in the middle, and the Upper Back is found inferiorly. The reader is encouraged to experiment with these locations and to gain his or her own clinical experience. I prefer the locations of *Chinese Acupuncture and Moxibustion.*

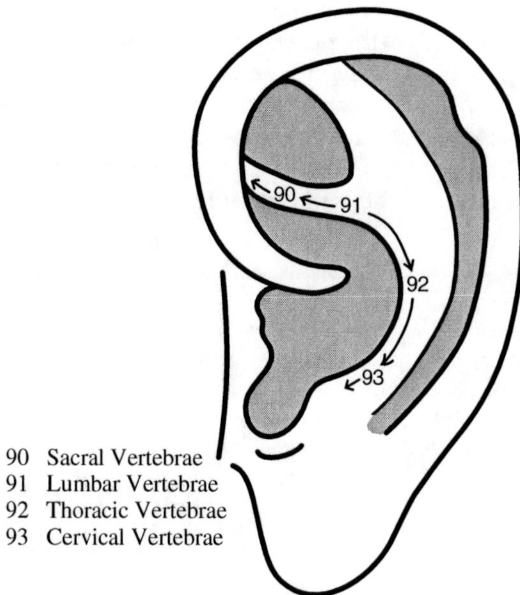

Figure 3.17 The vertebral points.

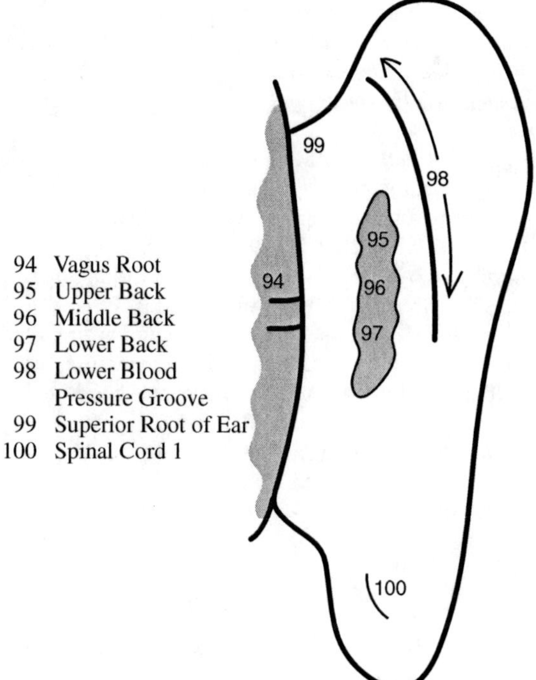

Figure 3.18 Points on the posterior aspect of the ear.

98. **Lower Blood Pressure Groove**: A groove-like depression on the back of the ear formed by the posterior border of the helix. It runs approximately the length of the upper third of the groove.
99. **Superior Root of the Ear**: Located on the posterior aspect of the ear at the intersection of the superior part of the auricle with the face.
100. **Spinal Cord 1**: Located on the posterior aspect of the ear at the superior border of the inferior annicular root.

References

1. Liu, H. *Auricular Diagnosis, Treatment, and Health Preservation*. Science Press, Beijing, China, 1996, p. 20.
2. Oleson, T. and Kroening, R. A comparison of Chinese and Nogier auricular acupuncture points. *Am. J. Acupunc.*, Jul.–Sept., 1983, 3: 206–222.
3. Hecker, H.U. *Color Atlas of Acupuncture: Body Points, Ear Points, Trigger Points.* Hippocrates, Stuttgart, Germany, 2001, p. 159.

Bibliography

Falk, C.X., Birch, S., Avants, S.K., Tsau, Y., and Margolin, A. Preliminary results of a new method for locating auricular acupuncture points. *Acupunc. Electrother. Res.*, 2000, 25(3–4): 165–177.

Foreign Language Press. *Chinese Acupuncture and Moxibustion*. Xinnong, C. (Ed.), Foreign Languages Press, Beijing, China, 1987.

Hecker, H.U. *Color Atlas of Acupuncture: Body Points, Ear Points, Trigger Points.* Hippocrates, Stuttgart, Germany, 2001.

Liu, H. *Auricular Diagnosis, Treatment, and Health Preservation.* Science Press, Beijing, China, 1996.

Nogier, P. *Handbook of Auriculotherapy.* Maisonneuve, Moulins-les–Metz, France, 1981.

Oleson, T.D., Kroening, R.J., and Bresler, D.E. An experimental evaluation of auricular diagnosis: the somatotopic mapping of musculoskeletal pain at ear acupuncture points. *Pain*, 1980, 8(2): 217–219.

Oleson, T. and Kroening, R. A comparison of Chinese and Nogier auricular acupuncture points. *Am. J. Acupunc.*, 1983, Jul.–Sept., 3: 206–222.

Omura, Y. New simple early diagnostic methods using Omura's "Bi–Digital O–Ring Dysfunction Localization method" and acupuncture organ representation points and their applications to the "drug and food compatibility test" for individual organs and to auricular diagnosis of internal organs: Part I. *Acupunc. Electrother. Res.*, 1981, 6(4): 239–254.

Shanghai, V. *College of Traditional Chinese Medicine. Acupuncture, a Comprehensive Text,* Bensley, D. and O'Conner, J. (trans./Ed.), Eastand Press, Seattle, WA, 1981.

Zhou, L. Supplementary comments on the standardization of auricular points. *J. Trad. Chin. Med.*, Jun. 18, 1995, 15(2): 132–134.

chapter four

The clinical energetics of the ear points

Objectives

- To understand the criteria for ear acupuncture point selection in a treatment
- To become familiar with the most common clinical energetics of the 100 common points of the ear consistent with the criteria for point selection

Introduction

Each ear point has numerous clinical applications. The clinical energetics described in this chapter are the physiological functions of those points that are traditionally recognized as consistent with Oriental medical theory. They are augmented with the thoughts of various ear acupuncture experts where relevant. These are the identical energetics that I have found effective in treating a wide variety of human illnesses. Because of the number of possible human health disorders, it is impossible to list all of the potential clinical usages of each point, nor is it necessary to do so. Each practitioner is encouraged to study these energetics so that he too can deduce any additional indications that might be possible based upon his understanding of Oriental medicine functions and the criteria for point selection as described. This deduction process likewise frees the practitioner from the memorization of point usage and an over reliance upon consulting texts so that he can be an efficient practitioner. The practitioner is encouraged to test his own hypotheses as well, concerning the use of ear points in order to gain his own clinical experience.

In auricular acupuncture, as well as in body acupuncture, points have many parameters for selection. Points can be selected based upon the following criteria:

- Western anatomical equivalent (i.e., the diseased area, organ, body part, or system) — for example, the Lung point could be chosen to treat a physical problem with the anatomical organ of the Lungs, such as constricted bronchioles.
- Western physiological counterpart — the Lung point could also be selected for a physiological problem of the Lung, such as edema of the Lungs.
- Anatomical equivalent in Oriental medicine — in Oriental medicine, the Lung point is useful for an anatomical Lung problem, such as invasion of the Lung by Wind–Cold.
- Physiological equivalent in Oriental medicine — an Oriental physiological Lung problem, such as failure of the Lungs to descend and disperse the fluids, is treated through the Lung point.
- Known clinical efficacy (i.e., as in the case of clinically effective points derived from clinical practice and research) — the Lung points, for instance, are clinically effective points in the treatment of Stomach ulcers because the Lungs dominate the mucous membranes. Ulcers are perforations of an organ's lining that consist of mucous membranes.
- Observation of morphological or pathological changes (i.e., pore-like depressions, creases, ridges, red areas, etc.) — red petechiae on a Lung point indicate Heat in the Lungs. The Lung point can treat this problem.
- Internal and external meridian pathways as well as other Oriental diagnostic paradigms that the practitioner may use (i.e., Five Elements, Triple Burner, Four Levels, Six Divisions, Three Treasures) — for instance, certain shoulder problems can be treated through the Lung point because the Lung meridian passes through the supraclavicular region of the shoulder area.

This guide assists the practitioner in thinking beyond merely selecting points based upon a simple anatomical equivalent of where the problem resides.

Oriental medicine's strength lies in its rich theory to meet the challenges of diagnosing and treating illness. Thoroughness, sensitivity, and creativity on the part of the practitioner in point selection enhance its effectiveness. For instance, most illness can be categorized according to Chinese medical theory under the 11 *Zang-fu* organs (with the Pericardium considered to be part of the Heart system). Hence, each organ can be the source of thousands of diseases. The ear points then have a wide range of clinical applicability that supercedes their Western equivalent organ or body part.

Because most points in the ear are named either according to a body part (i.e., Shoulder point), or according to an organ in a body system (i.e., the Stomach point), this simple nomenclature has allowed other healthcare providers, such as allopathic doctors, chiropractors, and researchers, to employ the ear diagnostically and therapeutically. However, without deeper understanding of Oriental medical theory, research studies about the clinical utility of an ear point can be flawed. For instance, in a scientific study that is designed to establish the relationship of one variable to another, a conclusion may be drawn that "X" point does not help in the treatment of a particular disease and, therefore, ear acupuncture is not effective in the treatment of that disorder. The "X" point may be the wrong point associated with the most effective treatment of the condition.

For instance, the Stomach point can help in the treatment of Stomach ulcers because the Stomach point focuses the treatment in the area of the Stomach. However, the Lung point is critical to the treatment of Stomach ulcers because the Lung dominates mucus membranes, and the ulcer is a problem with the mucus membranes of the Stomach. The choice of the Lung point for the treatment of Stomach ulcers is based on an appreciation of the Oriental physiological role of the Lungs. The treatment of Stomach ulcers is greatly enhanced through the addition of the Lung point as well. A Western study could conclude that ulcers are not effectively treated through ear acupuncture if the Lung point is not chosen.

Points of the triangular fossa

1. ***Shenmen***: I tend to think of ear *Shenmen* (translated as Spirit Gate) as energetically equivalent to Heart 7, *Shenmen*, in the body. In Oriental medicine, the Spirit is stored in the Heart. Like Heart 7, the Earth point of the Heart meridian, ear *Shenmen* has similar energetics in terms of grounding, balancing, and anchoring the Spirit. Therefore, *Shenmen* quiets the Heart, calms the Spirit, and puts the patient into a state of receptivity for treatment. Because of these energetics, *Shenmen* should be the first point treated in the ear for almost every ear prescription, with exceptions explored latter in the discussion of *Shenmen*.

   In Oriental medicine, the Heart dominates the mind and *Shenmen* fulfills this function. *Shenmen* can be used to treat those problems pertaining to the Heart in Oriental medicine, such as insomnia, dream-disturbed sleep, palpitations, tightness in the chest, angina, and memory and concentration problems. Any Heart problem from both a Western or an Oriental perspective, with the exception of the contraindicated conditions, benefits from treatment with *Shenmen*. Because of this connection to the mind, *Shenmen* is also a major point used in detoxification protocols for the symptoms of addiction withdrawal, such as restlessness and anxiety and the treatment of anxiety in general. "*Shenmen* has consistently been found as a core point in weight loss protocols for the same reasons."[1] (Anxiety and restlessness are common symptoms associated with the process of weight loss.)

   Shenmen is also a primary point for pain treatment. The *Neijing* (the *Yellow Emperor's Classic of Internal Medicine*, 500 to 300 B.C.) says, "When the Heart is serene, all pain is negligible." It should be an integral point in any pain prescription and, indeed, can function in this way. It is oftentimes the key point in a pain management plan.

   Because the Heart in Oriental medicine is connected to the eye system by way of its internal pathway, *Shenmen* is of benefit in the treatment of opthamological diseases. *Shenmen* is a primary point to reduce excess heat or inflammation. As such, it is a major point used to stop skin itching or breakouts that are often attributed to Heat in the Heart or Heat in the Blood because the Heart dominates the Blood. **Note/Contraindications**: The doctors with whom I studied in Beijing claim that the only contraindications for *Shenmen* are congestive heart failure and bronchitis characterized by excess phlegm, not phlegm or dampness that may be part of other health disorders. The reason why *Shenmen* is contraindicated for these conditions is because, as a point with Earth energetics, it has a dampening effect. Stimulating *Shenmen* adds Dampness to these already serious illnesses characterized by Damp. Therefore, the aforementioned conditions could become exacerbated and even more life threatening if *Shenmen* is used. Because of these cautions, I have not used *Shenmen* in the ear to treat congestive heart failure or bronchitis with excess phlegm, but have selected other points for treatment with as much success as can be expected for these complicated problems. In my opinion it would be negligent to ignore those admonitions from ones who are more knowledgeable than myself where there could be a possible risk to the health of the patient.

2. **Stop Wheezing**: This is a primary point for the treatment of wheezing that accompanies asthma, bronchitis, emphysema, and other respiratory or cardiovascular conditions. The Stop Wheezing point is especially effective when combined with the *Dingchuan* point in the ear, which also stops wheezing, and any of the Sympathetic points, which increase vasodilation and, thus, improve respiration.
3. **Hypertension**: Hypertension is an effective point to lower high blood pressure. If the variety of hypertension is due to *Yang* rising with True Heat manifestations vs. hypertension due to several other etiologies, bleeding the Hypertension point is particularly effective. Hypertension point works synergistically with the ear points (*Shenmen*, Liver, Heart, and the Lower Blood Pressure Groove) to reduce high blood pressure.

4.,5.,6. **Sympathetic**: Sympathetic is another point like *Shenmen* used to treat multiple conditions. It is directly related to the regulation of the nervous system.

The autonomic nervous system is made up of sympathetic and parasympathetic branches. Joseph Helms writes that the auricle displays the only external manifestation of the vagus nerve and thereby allows access to the functions of the autonomic nervous system.[2] The vagus nerve connects with the larynx, bronchii, heart, pancreas, liver, kidneys, and intestines. It exerts a direct influence on the regulation of stress.

The sympathetic branch corresponds to stress, flight, and fright reactions. Thus, the Sympathetic point when tonified stimulates the dilation of the blood vessels. Because of this ability, it is considered a primary point for pain since certain types of pain, such as fixed, stabbing, boring pain, in Oriental medicine is considered caused by constriction or Blood Stagnation, which results in pain.

The parasympathetic branch of the autonomic nervous system governs everyday organ functioning. When the sympathetic branch is dominant, the parasympathetic branch is suppressed. Sedating the Sympathetic point will assist in balancing both branches of the nervous system

Stimulation of this point causes the *Qi* energy to irrigate the cerebral meninges so that the point can be used to treat shock, trauma, and any nervous system disorder.

7. **Uterus/Prostate (Seminal Vesicle)**: This point can be used for all types of reproductive problems in both genders. Gynecological disorders, such as dysmenorrhea, amenorrhea, pelvic inflammatory disease, uterine cysts, fibroid tumors, and infertility, are treated with this point. For men, this point can be used to relieve swelling or contracture of the scrotum, and for testicular pain and prostate problems.
8. **Constipation**: This point can relieve constipation and impacted stools. It can be used to manage diverticulitis, diverticulosis, and sluggish bowels.
9. **Hepatitis**: This is one of several hepatitis points found in the ear, including point H 44. The Hepatitis point helps with the treatment of hepatitis when used along with the Liver, Spleen, and other Hepatitis points located in the ear.
10. **Hip Joint**: This point effectively relieves hip joint pain due to various etiologies.

Points of the lobe

11. **Upper Tooth**: This point can be used for dull, persistent, or painful toothache of the upper teeth. When stimulated with an electrical apparatus, the Upper Tooth point can be used to anesthetize the upper teeth.
12. **Tongue**: This point treats diseases of the tongue, such as tongue ulcerations or cancer, speech problems involving the tongue, such as aphasia, dysphasia, stuttering, or a deviated tongue that may be a sequel to stroke.
13. **Jaw:** This point can be used for problems with the jaw, such as clicking, tempromandibular joint syndrome, and an achy or dislocated jaw.
14. **Lower Tooth**: Similar to Upper Tooth point, Lower Tooth point treats the lower teeth. Lower Tooth can also be used as part of an acupuncture anesthesia protocol with electrical stimulation for lower tooth problems.
15. **Eye:** In the ear, this is the primary point to treat problems of the eye, such as decreased nighttime vision, eyestrain, declining vision, my-

opia, presbyopia, eye twitching, and many other opthamological disorders. The Eye point is especially effective when combined with other ear points, such as Eye 1 and 2, Brain, Heart, Liver, Spleen, and *Shenmen* whose energetics also relate to the health of the eye. In China, Eye point is used to treat teenage myopia with good success.

16. **Inner Ear**: This point is for problems of the inner ear, such as impaired hearing, tinnitus, Meniere's syndrome, problems of balance, and motion sickness (i.e., vertigo, seasickness, and inner ear infection). The energetics of Inner Ear are similar to the body acupuncture point, Pericardium 6 (*Neiguan*) in regard to balance.
17. **Helix 5**: Like all the Helix points, Helix 5 enhances immunity.
18. **Tonsil**: Tonsil pertains to tonsillar tissue, especially the palatine tonsils in the throat, which ward off infection. Tonsil can be used to treat tonsillitis.
19. **Helix 6**: The energetics of Helix 6 are similar to point #17, Helix 5. These points influence immunity.
20. **Insomnia**: Insomnia can promote sleep if the point is rubbed gently.

Note: This point may have the opposite effect if stimulated too vigorously.

Points of the tragus

21. **Thirst**: The Thirst point can regulate thirst whether if it is excessive or insufficient. The Thirst point is commonly used in weight loss protocols to reduce fluid consumption.
22. **External Nose**: Primarily used for problems on the exterior of the nose; External Nose treats acne, broken blood vessels of the nose, and rhinitis.
23. **Hunger**: Depending upon which acupuncture technique is used, the Hunger point can reduce or stimulate hunger. Hunger is traditionally used as part of weight loss or stop smoking protocols where there is a tendency to satisfy oral cravings by eating.
24. **Internal Nose**: Internal Nose, as its name implies, treats problems such as runny nose, stuffy nose, sinus pressure, maxillary sinusitis, polyps, and bloody nose.
25. **Adrenal**: Adrenal point is a major point for treating shock, pulselessness, asthma, hypotension, stress, infection, inflammation, and trauma. Adrenal regulates adrenal hormones and treats cough and shortness of breath due to adrenal insufficiency.

Points of the scaphoid fossa

26. **Wrist**: This point treats wrist problems, such as arthritis, sprains, strains or breaks, contracture of the wrist, carpal tunnel syndrome, and arthritis.

27. **Fingers**: This point can be treated for spasm, contracture, swelling, and arthritis of the fingers as well as other problems of the fingers.
28. **Allergy**: Allergy point can be used for various allergies, such as respiratory or food allergies, multiple chemical sensitivities, or for patients with weakened immune systems.
29. **Shoulder**: Shoulder point is a clinically effective point to treat shoulder problems. It can be used to treat shoulder pain, tight shoulders, impaired shoulder mobility, frozen shoulder, rotator cuff disorders, and other shoulder disorders.
30. **Elbow**: This point can treat elbow problems, such as golfer's elbow, tennis elbow, carpenter's elbow, and other elbow joint disorders.
31. **Clavicle**: The clavicle point can be used in treating a broken clavicle, extra bone growth on the clavicle, or other problems involving the clavicle.
32. **Shoulder Joint**: This point can be used similarly to the Shoulder point especially if the problem (i.e., bursitis, synovitis) is more confined to the shoulder joint vs. the musculature of the shoulder.
33. **Thyroid**: Thyroid is excellent for regulating the thyroid gland as in cases of hypothyroidism or hyperthyroidism.
34. **Nephritis**: The Nephritis point is used to treat inflammation of the Kidneys.

Points of the cavum concha

35. **Mouth**: The mouth point can be used to increase or decrease appetite. It is commonly used along with point #20, Hunger, in weight loss and stop smoking protocols to reduce both appetite and oral fixation. The Mouth point is also referred to as "the Antifatigue point." Because the Mouth point is located in a very tender area of the ear, stimulating the Mouth point is invigorating. This factor accounts for the point's effectiveness in counteracting fatigue. Additionally, Mouth point stimulates appetite or the desire for food. The increase in fuel that comes from food consumption increases energy. This point can also be used to treat mouth problems, such as ulcers, canker sores, and deviation of the mouth. Mouth point can also have an invigorating effect if a dispersion technique is applied, so be aware that the Mouth point is contraindicated when one is treating fatigue that accompanies insomnia as it can keep the patient awake.
36. **Heart**: This point can be used for all Heart problems in both Oriental and Western diagnosis. Western diagnostic conditions would include tightness in the chest, palpitations, angina, circulation problems, hypertension, mitral valve prolapse, and stroke. Chinese diagnostic problems include all of the above as well as memory and concentration problems, emotional problems, anxiety, restlessness, and psychological disturbances, easy daytime sweat, and insomnia.

Because the Heart is the Supreme Controller in Oriental medicine and moves the *Qi* and the Blood, the Heart point can also be used to control pain by moving Stagnant *Qi* and Blood in the body. Heart point is also effective in treating eye problems because in Oriental medicine the Heart has an internal pathway or "eye system" that runs from the Heart to the eye.

37. **Trachea**: This point treats breathing, cough, constriction of the throat, speech problems, and other problems of the trachea.
38. **Upper Lung**: Upper Lung is essential in all respiratory problems, such as shortness of breath, asthma, bronchitis, swollen glands, common cold, flu, and sore throat. From the Chinese perspective, Lung is the master of the *Qi*. Therefore, Upper Lung is a primary point for increasing energy and moving the *Qi*. This is the identical reason why it has been found clinically to be the major point in withdrawal symptoms because it improves and regulates systemic energy thereby contributing to a feeling of well being.

    Some sources say, the Upper Lung point corresponds to the opposite Lung (contralateral lung), and the Lower Lung point corresponds to the Lung on the same side of the body as the ear (ipsilateral lung). For instance, when looking at the left ear of a patient, the Upper Lung point corresponds to the right lung and the Lower Lung point corresponds to the left lung. I do not use them as pertaining to the right or the left sides.
39. **Lower Lung**: Lower Lung can be used similarly to Upper Lung to enhance Lung function. It can be selected if the patient needs to breathe more deeply or if the patient's problem is in the lower part of the Lung. I use it this way, as well as when ear pathology is present on this point or to reinforce the action of the Upper Lung.

    Some sources suggests, you may use the Lower Lung point in the ear to treat the Lung on the same side of the body as the side of the ear being treated; that is, select the Lower Lung point in the left ear to treat the left lung and the Lower Lung point in the right ear to treat the right lung.

Note: The Lung points are sometimes called the Dermis points. They are major dermatological points for urticaria, reducing inflammation and irritation of the skin and mucous membranes, and promoting healing because the Lung dominates the skin and mucus membranes. This includes the internal mucus membranes of the mouth, nose, throat, stomach, and other locations. As a result, Lung points are primary, clinically effective points for stomach and duodenal ulcers, ulcerative colitis, and other internal abrasions.

40. **Esophagus**: The Esophagus point is used for treating difficulty in swallowing, acid reflux disease (esophageal reflux), acid regurgitation, and other esophageal problems.

41. **Cardiac Sphincter**: This is a very powerful point used to regulate the cardiac sphincter, which is the upper orifice of the stomach. If the sphincter is incompetent, acid from the stomach can enter the esophagus and lead to acid reflux disease.
42. **Stomach**: This point treats Stomach ulcers, gastralgia, dyspepsia, vomiting, nausea, and other Stomach problems. According to Oriental medicine, the Stomach assists in the rottening and ripening of the food, thus contributing to the formation of *Qi* and Blood. The Stomach point resolves Dampness and Phlegm. It is used in weight loss protocols to reduce appetite. *Shenmen* and the Lung points have also been found to be core points in treating weight problems for the reasons discussed above.
43. **Liver**: Liver is an important ear point used for all clinical energetics pertaining to the Liver in Chinese medicine. Liver point is used to move *Qi* Stagnation and Blood Stagnation, build Blood, and nourish *Yin*. Treating the Liver point benefits the eyes, tendons, muscles, ligaments, and nerves. It is a major point for facilitating digestion and for regulating hormonal and menstrual function. It treats stress, depression, migraines, hepatitis, spasm, convulsions, pain, and other symptoms that are a result of Liver dysfunction.
44. **Hepatitis**: This Hepatitis point, located within the cavum concha, specifically within the Liver area, is an additional point that can be used to treat the difficult disease of hepatitis that is common in China as well as a rising health problem throughout the world.
45. **Relax Muscle**: This point, located within the Liver area, is especially good for encouraging muscular relaxation. Pain comes from stagnation and stagnation can lead to muscular tension. Therefore, Relax Muscle is an important point for relieving pain. Relax muscle is a central point in any pain treatment strategy for muscular pain, such as menstrual cramps or back pain. Relax Muscle is also good for tension and relaxation in general. Like Gallbladder 34 (*Yanglinguan*) in the body (the Influential Point that dominates the Muscles), Relax Muscle is an auricular point that treats muscular pain.
46. **Spleen**: This point can be used to treat any Spleen syndrome in Oriental medicine, such as Spleen *Qi* and *Yang* deficiency, or Spleen *Qi* Deficiency with Repletion of Dampness, Blood production, problems of the muscles, abdominal distention, and lethargy. The Spleen point assists in the production of white blood cells, thereby enhancing immune function. The Spleen point is an important point in the regulation of digestion, assuming the function of absorption of food that is assigned to the Small Intestine in Western medicine.
47. ***Sanjiao* (Triple Warmer)**: This point connects all three *Jiaos*. In Oriental medicine, the Triple Warmer assists in the regulation of water passageways such that the *Sanjiao* point eliminates excess Water or Damp, thereby treating edema. *Sanjiao* is also the theoretical construct used

to explain the production of *Qi*, Blood, and body fluid that become the Essential Substances (*Qi*, Blood, *Jinye*). Thus, the *Sanjiao* point facilitates digestion and distributes the Essential Substances to the entire body. In this way the *Sanjiao* point strengthens immunity and can be used to fight off exogenous evils. The point also treats constipation.

Interestingly, clinical studies have found it to be an effective point for relaxation, and in the treatment of anxiety and psychosomatic disorders.[3]

Points of the cymba concha

48. **Duodenum**: This point is for problems of the duodenum, such as a duodenal ulcer. The Duodenum point stimulates the absorptive aspects of digestion.
49. **Small Intestine**: This point can be used to treat problems of the Small Intestine, such as digestive disturbances, particularly food absorption problems. Small Intestine point aids in the separation of the "pure from the impure." Small Intestine point can be used for treating urinary tract infections due to "Heat in the Heart shifting to the Small Intestine" because the Heart is the coupled organ of the Small Intestine. For the same reason, Small Intestine point can also treat palpitations.
50. **Large Intestine**: The Large Intestine point can regulate the Large Intestine and help with problems such as water absorption, loose stools, diarrhea and/or constipation, hemorrhoids, irritable bowel syndrome, and ulcerative colitis.
51. **Appendix**: This point is useful in treating inflammation of the vermiform appendix as in acute simple appendicitis.
52. **Bladder**: The Bladder point is for treating problems, such as frequency of urination, dribbling urination, urinary incontinence, urinary urgency, difficult urination, painful urination, enuresis, retention of urine, stones, bladder infections, cloudy urination, and other urinary problems.
53. **Kidney**: The Kidney point can be utilized to treat a vast array of disorders that are considered Kidney diseases in Oriental medicine. Such disorders include problems connected with Bladder function, with the foundation *Yin* and *Yang*, and growth, maturation, and development. The Kidney point is an important point in respiratory disorders because in Oriental medicine the Kidney grasps the *Qi* of the Lungs. This point treats immune disorders, builds Blood, and regulates body warmth. It can be used for kidney stones, nephritis, lumbago, tinnitus, and other Kidney problems.
54. **Ureters**: This point treats stones (also called kidney stones) that have collected in the ureters, and assists in the elimination of urine.
55. **Pancreas/Gallbladder**: This point assists in sugar/insulin regulation and promotes proper bile flow. It participates in the breakdown

of fats and helps the Liver in its *Yang* functions. It treats cholecystitis, cholelithiasis, pancreatitis, diseases of the bile duct, gallstones, diabetes, and other problems of the Gallbladder and Pancreas. Dr. James Yin Tau So claims that the Pancreas point is found in the left ear and the Gallbladder point in the right."[4] Sometimes the Pancreas point is called the Diabetes point. I treat both the pancreas and the gallbladder equally through each ear.

Points of the helix

56. **Diaphragm**: The Diaphragm point is a powerful point that triggers movement of the diaphragm, thus assisting in deep breathing. According to traditional Oriental medical theory, the diaphragm is the place where the Blood meets and then is directed to its proper pathways. Therefore, the Diaphragm point is effective in the treatment of *Qi* and Blood Stagnation. It is indicated for diseases caused by bleeding due to Evil Heat in the Blood. When the diaphragm moves, Liver *Qi* is regulated and spread, and the distribution of *Qi* and *Blood* in the *Upper Jiao* is facilitated.

    The Diaphragm point also has an effect upon the emotions by virtue of moving Liver *Qi* Stagnation. Consequently, it treats depression viewed as Liver *Qi* stagnation, and regularizes the emotions. This point then helps the *Upper Jiao* and the *Middle Jiao* communicate, and dispels chest and mid-back tightness. Because it corresponds to the diaphragm, this point is good for treating nervous tension, hiccups, and pressure from the Stomach or Liver that follows surgery. It also treats jaundice.

    This point has mixed sympathetic/parasympathetic innervations. Kropej recommends needling it first in a treatment because it affects the reactive ability of the rest of the auricle. He says that it can make an unreactive ear reactive or a hypersensitive ear normal because it promotes homeostatic control. The Diaphragm point also corresponds to the umbilical area.[5] Some say this point does not correspond to the body's anatomy. They have delineated its role based upon a functional observation of its effects.[6] Some authors refer to this point as Point Zero (Nogier) or the Master point (Oleson).
57. **Lower portion of the rectum**: This point remedies problems, such as fecal stagnation, constipation, impacted stools, hemorrhoids, diverticulitis, and diverticuloses of the lower rectum.
58. **Hemorrhoids**: This is a point specifically for the treatment of hemorrhoids due to Stagnant Blood, Damp-heat accumulation, or prolapsed *Qi*. It also treats itchiness, inflammation, local bleeding, and anal fissures.
59. **Common Cold**: This point can be used to help prevent the common cold or to treat a developed cold. It can be used for symptoms of

Wind–Cold, Wind–Heat, or Wind–Dampness that cause common cold manifestations.

60. **Ear Apex**: This is an important point to bring down *Yang* and reduce heat. In the case of *Yang* rising, this point reduces high blood pressure and can quell anger and other heat manifestations symptomatic of *Yang* rising. Especially when a bleeding technique is used, it is a clinically effective point for conjunctivitis, migraines, and other symptoms of Liver *Yang* rising.

61., 62., 63., 64. **Helixes 1 to 4**: Because these points pertain to tonsillar tissue, they can be used to enhance immunity and ward off infection or invasion, such as acute tonsillitis.

Points of the antitragus

65. ***Dingchuan***: Analogous to the body point *Dingchuan* on the back of the neck (0.5 cun lateral to GV 14 – *Dazhui*), this is another very powerful point to assist in stop wheezing. It is excellent for bronchitis, asthma, and other breathing difficulties. *Dingchuan* is sometimes called the Ear asthma point. It works well with the Stop Wheezing point located in the triangular fossa.
66. **Brain (also known as Subcortex)**: The Brain point is involved in regulating the excitation and inhibition of the cerebral cortex. Diseases of the nervous, digestive, endocrine, and uritogenital systems, as well as hemorrhage, insomnia, inflammation, pain, swelling, shock, prolapse, and excessive sweating can be treated with this point. In my opinion, Brain point is the second most important point in the ear, with *Shenmen* being first. I use it to augment almost every treatment because the brain controls every bodily activity. According to some sources, the Brain point corresponds to the pituitary gland.
67. **Occiput**: To treat the occiput locally in cases such as occipital headache, dizziness, neck tension, stiffness along the nape, or Blood Stasis patterns in the occipital area, use the Occiput point. Because the visual cortex of the brain is located in the occiput, this point can be used to treat a multitude of eye disorders. Occiput also treats neuropsychiatric disorders, psychosis, pain, shock, inflammation, convulsions, lockjaw, and regulates the nervous system. In addition, it can be used to relieve motion sickness.
68. **Temple**: This is a local point for treating problems of the temple, such as breakouts, tension, temporal headaches, one-sided headaches, and migraines. It is sometimes called the *Taiyang* point because body acupuncture point *Taiyang* is located at the temple.
69. **Forehead:** This point is useful for treating local problems of the forehead, such as wrinkles, acne, and pain and congestion of the sinuses and/or forehead. It is used to treat *Yangming* (Large Intestine/Stomach) headaches.

70. **Brainstem**: This point treats disorders of the cerebral blood vessels and meninges, incomplete development of the brain, apoplexy, convulsions, and stiffness along the nape, sequel to cerebral shock, and respiration.

71., 72. **Eye 1 and Eye 2**: These are supplemental points used in remedying a wide array of eye disorders, such as glaucoma and myopia. Use with the Eye point on the lobe (#15) as the primary point in the formula; supplement with Liver, Heart, Spleen, and Stomach ear points. The Spleen and Stomach process nutrients for the body that creates the blood. Blood is necessary for eye health and sight.

73. **Raise Blood Pressure**: This point can raise blood pressure and, as such, it is useful in emergency situations in which the blood pressure needs to be raised.
74. **Ovaries/Testes:** This point can be used to treat a variety of reproductive disorders involving the ovaries in women or the testes in men, including irregular menstruation and infertility.
75. **Endocrine (also called the Internal Secretion point)**: This point is used to regulate all endocrine secretions in the body; thus, it is useful for hormonal problems.

Points of the antihelix

76. **Toe**: For diverse toe problems, such as fractures, bunions, hammertoes, arthritis, and other traumatic disorders, this point can be used.
77. **Heel**: This point can be used for heel problems, such as calcaneal spurs.
78. **Ankle**: This point is for ankle problems, such as breaks, sprains, and swelling.
79. **Knee**: Knee is a key point for a variety of knee problems, such as knee crepitation, achiness, weakness, cold knees, disorders involving knee ligaments or the knee joint, or for circulation problems around the knee.
80. **Lumbago**: This is an excellent, clinically effective point for low back pain in the lumbar region. This used to be the old Knee point in earlier literature. Now the Knee area is above the Lumbago point.
81. **Sciatic Nerve**: Another quick acting, clinically effective point, Sciatic Nerve treats symptoms of a compressed sciatic nerve and radiating pain down the back of the leg.
82. **Ischium**: The Ischium point treats problems originating from the buttocks, such as sciatica or problems pertaining to the ischium, and the lower portion of the hipbone.
83. **Buttocks**: The Buttocks point can also be used to treat the ischium or other gluteal problems.
84. **Abdomen**: The abdomen area is good for treating general, diffuse, or specific abdominal problems. It can be used alone or for reinforce-

ment in combination with a point for a specific part of the abdomen, such as the Large Intestine point or the Appendix point.

85. **Chest**: This point treats a vast array of chest problems, such as tightness in the chest, shortness of breath, asthma, cough, cold, and other respiratory or chest disorders. Like the Abdomen point, the Chest point can be used singularly or in combination with other points in the region of the problem, such as the Mammary points, Lung, Heart, etc.

86., 87. **Mammary Glands**: These two points are excellent for the treatment of fibrocystic breast disease, breast distention, and tenderness.

88. **Neck**: The Neck point is a fast-working point for treating a host of neck problems, among them stiff neck, torticollis, cervical disease, and misaligned vertebrae.

89. **Throat/Teeth**: This point treats throat or teeth problems, such as tonsillitis, sore throat, and constriction in the throat, or teeth problems in general.

90., 92., 93. **The Spinal Points: Sacral, Lumbar, Thoracic, and Cervical Vertebrae**: Each group of points pertains to a particular segment of the spinal column. These are superb points especially effective for adjusting the vertebrae in the associated portion of the spinal cord. Additionally, they can be used to treat the nerves originating from the correlating portions of the spinal cord, that innervate the organs and the dermatomal areas.

Points on the posterior aspect of the ear

94. **Vagus**: This is a strong point to regulate functions and organs of the *Middle Jiao*, which is where the vagus nerve largely supplies. The Vagus point is used to treat digestive disorders like gastralgia and helps expel gallstones. It is also good for remedying headaches, asthma, stomachaches, palpitations, bowel problems, and any areas that the vagus nerve, the longest cranial nerve in the body, innervates.

95., 96., 97. **Upper, Middle, and Lower Back**: These points correspond to a variety of back problems. For added reinforcement, it is helpful to use these points with the corresponding back points on the front of the ear; for instance, use Upper Back on the back of the ear with Upper Thoracic Vertebrae on its anterior surface.

98. **Lower Blood Pressure Groove**: This is a powerful groove used to lower high blood pressure, especially when the groove is bled.

99. **Superior Root of the Ear**: This point treats hemiplegia.

100. **Spinal Cord 1**: This point can be used to treat muscular atrophy and paralysis.

Table 4.1 summarizes the location of each point discussed herein along with their major clinical energetics.

Table 4.1 Auricular Acupuncture Points: Location and Energetics

Point	Ear Zone	Specific Location	Energetics
#1 *Shenmen*	Triangular Fossa	In the triangular fossa, along the lateral border, superior to the junction of its inferior and superior borders. **Tip:** Put your ear probe into this juncture and then slide superiorly to it. You will fall into a small depression; that is the point.	Quiets the Heart, calms the spirit, puts the patient into a state of receptivity for treatment. Reduces inflammation. First point for almost every treatment. Heart problems such as insomnia, dream disturbed sleep, palpitations, angina, memory and concentration problems, pain, opthamological diseases. Skin itching, detoxification, restlessness, anxiety, weight loss protocols. Contraindications: Congestive heart failure and bronchitis characterized by excess phlegm.
#2 Stop Wheezing	Triangular Fossa	In the deepest point in the center of the triangular fossa. **Tip:** Put your probe roughly in this vicinity; now search by feel for the depression which is where the point is located.	Wheezing accompanying asthma, bronchitis, or emphysema, or other respiratory or cardiovascular conditions. It is especially effective when combined with *Dingchuan* (in the ear) and one of the sympathetic points that increases vasodilation.

(*continued*)

Table 4.1 (continued). Auricular Acupuncture Points: Location and Energetics

Point	Ear Zone	Specific Location	Energetics
#3 Hypertension	Triangular Fossa	In the laterosuperior corner of the triangular fossa.	Hypertension It works synergistically with *Shenmen*, Liver, Heart, and the lower blood pressure groove.
#4 Sympathetic 1	Triangular Fossa	In the mediosuperior corner of the triangular fossa.	Balances the autonomic nervous system, nourishes *yin*, and dilates the blood vessels. Pain, shock, trauma, and any nervous system disorders.
#5 Sympathetic 2	Triangular Fossa	On the internal aspect of the helix midway between the level of Sympathetic 1 and Sympathetic 3.	
#6 Sympathetic 3	Triangular Fossa	On the inferior antihelix crus, below Sympathetic 1.	
#7 Uterus/Prostate (Seminal Vesicle)	Triangular Fossa	Midway between the Hypertension and Sympathetic 1 points, along the superior border of the triangular fossa.	Reproductive problems, gynecological disorders, such as dysmenorrhea, amenorrhea, pelvic inflammatory disease, uterine cysts, fibroid tumors, and infertility. Swelling or contracture of the scrotum, testicular pain, and infertility.

#8 Constipation	Triangular Fossa	On the inferior border of the triangular fossa. This point is an area equivalent to a rectangular shape. The upper part is along the inferior border of the triangular fossa and the lower part is on the upper portion of the inferior antihelix crus.	Constipation and impacted stools.
#9 Hepatitis	Triangular Fossa	At the junction of the inferior and superior borders of the triangular fossa.	It can help with the treatment of hepatitis along with the Liver, Spleen, and other Hepatitis points.
#10 Hip Joint	Triangular Fossa	Medial to the Hepatitis point, on the lower border of the triangular fossa.	Hip joint pain.
#11 Upper Teeth	Lobe	In the postero-inferior aspect of Sector 1.	Dull or persistent toothache of the upper teeth. Upper tooth extractions.
#12 Tongue	Lobe	In the center of Sector 2.	Tongue ulcerations, cancer, or other problems with the tongue, such as aphasia, dysphasia, stuttering, or a deviated tongue.
#13 Jaw	Lobe	In the center of Sector 3.	Jaw problems, such as clicking, tempromandibular joint syndrome, achy or dislocated jaw.

(*continued*)

Table 4.1 (continued). Auricular Acupuncture Points: Location and Energetics

Point	Ear Zone	Specific Location	Energetics
#14 Lower Teeth	Lobe	In the center of Sector 4.	This point can be used similarly to the Upper Tooth point except that this is for the lower teeth.
#15 Eye	Lobe	In the center of Sector 5.	Problems of the eye, such as decreased nighttime vision, eyestrain, declining vision, myopia, presbyopia, eye twitching, and a host of opthamological disorders. It is especially effective when combined with Eye 1 and Eye 2, Brain, Heart, Liver, Spleen, and *Shenmen*.
#16 Inner Ear	Lobe	In the center of Sector 6.	This point is for problems of the inner ear, such as impaired hearing, tinnitus, Meniere's syndrome, problems of balance and motion sickness, such as vertigo and seasickness.
#17 Helix 5	Lobe	On the lateral border of Sector 6.	Like all the Helix points, this point enhances immunity by strengthening tonsillar tissue.
#18 Tonsil	Lobe	In the center of Sector 8.	This point pertains to the tonsillar tissue, especially the palantine tonsils in the form of tonsillitis, which wards off infection.
#19 Helix 6	Lobe	On the lower margin of Sector 8.	This point's energetics are similar to point #17.

#20 Insomnia	Lobe	Slightly medial to the Teeth points on the horizontal line dividing the Upper Tooth and Lower Tooth points.	This point can promote sleep if rubbed gently. *Note:* It may have the opposite effect if stimulated too vigorously.
#21 Thirst	Tragus	In the center of the superior portion of the tragus.	Regulates thirst. It is commonly used in weight loss protocols.
#22 External Nose	Tragus	Midway between the Thirst and Hunger points in the center of the tragus.	Exterior nose problem, acne, broken blood vessels, and rhinitis.
#23 Hunger	Tragus	In the center of the tragus, at the level of its lower lobe directly below the External Nose point.	Regulates hunger; part of weight loss or stop smoking protocols.
#24 Internal Nose	Tragus	Midway between the Hunger and Adrenal points on the lower portion of the tragus.	Internal nose problems, polyps, runny nose, stuffy nose, sinus pressure, maxillary sinusitis, and bloody nose.
#25 Adrenal	Tragus	On the lower portion of the tragus, close to its lateral border.	Shock, stress, infection, inflammation, and trauma that depletes the adrenal glands. Regulates adrenal hormones, treats asthma and cough due to adrenal insufficiency. For hypotension and pulselessness.

(*continued*)

Table 4.1 (continued). Auricular Acupuncture Points: Location and Energetics

Point	Ear Zone	Specific Location	Energetics
#26 Wrist	Scaphoid Fossa	Opposite the tubercle of the helix.	Wrist problems, such as carpal tunnel syndrome, sprains, strains or breaks, contracture of the wrist.
#27 Finger	Scaphoid Fossa	In the uppermost portion of the scapha. **Tip:** Think of the Finger point as a bigger area. "I picture this area like the length of extended Fingers."	Spasm, contracture, swelling, arthritis of the fingers, and other finger problems.
#28 Allergy	Scaphoid Fossa	In the scapha, midway between the Wrist and Finger points.	Respiratory and food allergies, or multiple chemical sensitivities, weak immunity.
#29 Shoulder	Scaphoid Fossa	In the scapha, level with the crus of the helix.	The Shoulder point is one of the most clinically effective points to treat shoulder problems. It can be used for shoulder pain, tight shoulders, frozen shoulder, impaired mobility and rotator cuff disorders, and other shoulder disorders.
#30 Elbow	Scaphoid Fossa	In the scapha, midway between the Wrist and the Shoulder points.	This point can treat elbow problems, such as golfer's elbow, carpenter's elbow, and other elbow and joint disorders.

#31 Clavicle	Scaphoid Fossa	In the scapha, level with the height of the antitragus.	The Clavicle point can be used for a broken clavicle or extra bone growth on the clavicle, or other problems involving the clavicle.
#32 Shoulder Joint	Scaphoid Fossa	In the scapha, midway between the Shoulder and Clavicle points.	This point can be used similarly to the Shoulder, especially if the problem is more confined to the shoulder joint vs. those having muscular involvement.
#33 Thyroid	Scaphoid Fossa	On the medial border of the scapha, parallel but slightly inferior to the Throat and Teeth point (F 89).	This is one of several Thyroid points in the ear that is excellent for regulating the thyroid gland.
#34 Nephritis	Scaphoid Fossa	Below the Clavicle point, at the end of the lateral border of the scapha.	The Nephritis point can be used to treat inflammation of the Kidney.
#35 Mouth	Cavum Concha	This area, like a smile, parallels the lateral border of the external auditory meatus.	The Mouth point can be used to increase or decrease appetite. It is commonly used in weight loss and stop smoking protocols both to reduce appetite and oral fixation. It is also referred to as the Antifatigue point. Because it is located in a very tender area of the ear, this partly accounts for the effect of picking up energy. It stimulates appetite which, if satisfied, will usually lead to an increase in energy as well. It can also be used for mouth problems, such as ulcers, canker sores, facial paralysis, and other similar problems.

(*continued*)

Table 4.1 (continued). Auricular Acupuncture Points: Location and Energetics

Point	Ear Zone	Specific Location	Energetics
#36 Heart	Cavum Concha	At the deepest point of the cavum concha, at the level of the center of the Mouth point. **Tip:** Eyeball the area and then search with your probe for the deepest point.	This point can be treated for all Heart problems from both a TC and Western perspective. Such conditions would include angina, palpitations, mitral valve prolapse, tightness in the chest, circulation problems, hypertension, and stroke. Chinese differentiations would include memory and concentration problems, easy daytime sweat, insomnia, emotional problems, hysteria, anxiety, restlessness, and psychological disturbances. It can also be used to control pain by moving Stagnant *Qi* and Blood in the body because the Heart is the Supreme Controller. It is also effective for eye problems as well (see discussion under *Shenmen*) because the internal pathway of the Heart has an "eye system" that goes from the Heart to the eye.
#37 Trachea	Cavum Concha	A horizontal area that starts at the center of the Mouth point and extends to the Heart point.	This point can be used for cough, breathing, throat, and speech problems; constriction of the trachea and other problems of the trachea.

#38 Upper Lung	Cavum Concha	In the depression above the Heart point. **Tip:** Put your probe in the Heart point and then slide slightly above it until the probe falls into a depression.	Upper Lung can be used similarly to Lower Lung to enhance Lung function. It is called for in all respiratory problems, such as asthma, bronchitis, sore throat, swollen glands, common cold, flu, cough, asthma, and hemoptysis. Additionally, from the Chinese perspective because Lung is the Master of the *Qi*, this is a primary point for increasing energy and moving it. This is the identical reason as to why it has been clinically found to be the major point in withdrawal symptoms because it regulates systemic energy. It is a major dermatological point to reduce inflammation, irritation, and promote healing because the Lung dominates the skin and mucus membranes, which includes internal mucus membranes of the mouth, nose, throat, stomach, and others. It is a primary point for urticaria. As a result, it is a primary, clinically effective point for stomach and duodenal ulcers, ulcerative colitis, and other abrasions. According to Mario Wexu, the Upper Lung point corresponds to the opposite Lung and the Lower Lung point corresponds to the Lung on the same side of the body as the ear. This is also corroborated by Chinese clinical trials.[7]

(*continued*)

Table 4.1 (continued). Auricular Acupuncture Points: Location and Energetics

Point	Ear Zone	Specific Location	Energetics
#39 Lower Lung	Cavum Concha	In the depression below the Heart point. **Tip:** Put your probe on the Heart point and then slide slightly below it until the probe falls into a depression.	This point is used similarly to Upper Lung. It can be used if the patient needs to breathe deeper or if the patient's problem is in the lower part of the Lung. As Wexu says it can treat the Lung on the same side of the body as the side of the ear being treated.
#40 Esophagus	Cavum Concha	**Tip:** Take the length of the distance from the upper curvature of the Mouth to the lateral end of the lower border of the crus of the helix. Divide this distance in half. The most medial half is the Esophagus area.	The Esophagus point is used for difficulty in swallowing, acid reflux disease (esophageal reflux), acid regurgitation, and other esophageal problems.
#41 Cardiac Sphincter	Cavum Concha	The second lateral, half of the distance below the crus of the helix, which is found as described above.	This is a very powerful point used to regulate the cardiac sphincter, which is the upper orifice of the Stomach. If it is loose, acid from the stomach may enter the esophagus, leading to acid reflux disease.

#42 Stomach	Cavum Concha	A round area that begins at the end of the crus of the helix and extends halfway into the distance formed by the end of the crus and the medial border of the lower antihelix crus. **Tip:** Due to the pathology that can develop in the stomach area (discussed in Chapter 7), the best way to locate this point is as follows: Place your probe in the Diaphragm point (Point B 56). Slide off the crus of the helix into a little notch that you can feel with the probe. That point is the beginning of the Stomach area. The Stomach now extends half way across the area of the cymba/cavum concha in a circular manner. (See Figure 3.1.)	This point is for Stomach ulcers, gastralgia, dyspepsia, vomiting, nausea, and other local problems. Energetically, it assists in the rottening and ripening of the food, thus promoting the formation of *Qi* and Blood. It resolves Dampness and Phlegm.

(*continued*)

Table 4.1 (continued). Auricular Acupuncture Points: Location and Energetics

Point	Ear Zone	Specific Location	Energetics
#43 Liver	Cavum Concha	Comprises the second half of the distance from the Stomach to the medial border of the lower antihelix crus. It is roughly a triangular-shaped area. Its superior border is formed by a 45-degree angle from the upper border of the stomach to the medial border of the lower antihelix crus. Its lower border is level with the lower border of the crus of the helix.	Liver is a primary ear point used for all the major clinical energetics pertaining to Liver in Chinese medicine. It is used to move *Qi* Stagnation, Blood Stagnation, build Blood, and nourish *Yin*. It benefits the eyes, tendons, muscles, ligaments, and nerves, and is a primary point for facilitating digestion, and regulating hormonal and menstrual function.
#44 Hepatitis	Cavum Concha	Area found within the Liver area, close to the lateral curvature of the Stomach.	Here is another Hepatitis point located within the Liver area that can be used to treat this disorder.
#45 Relax Muscle	Cavum Concha	Within the Liver area. It is roughly a circular area, below the superior border of the Liver area.	This point, located within the Liver area, is especially good for assisting in muscular relaxation. As such, it becomes a primary point for pain because pain is stagnation and, as such, has a muscular component to it. It is a core point in a pain treatment strategy and applicable to many pain conditions. It is also good for tension and relaxation, in general.

#46 Spleen	Cavum Concha	This point is a large area. **Tip:** First locate the midpoint of the lower border of the Liver. Now, extend a line vertically downward to where it intersects superior to the antitragus.The area lateral to it is the Spleen area.	This point can be used for all the Spleen syndromes in Oriental medicine, such as Spleen *Qi* and *Yang* deficiency, Repletion with Dampness, Blood production, and problems of muscles. It assists in the production of white blood cells, thereby enhancing immunity. It is an important point in the regulation of digestion, abdominal distention, and lethargy.
#47 *Sanjiao*	Cavum Concha	In the deepest point of the cavum concha at the level of the intertragic notch. **Tip:** To locate this point, "look" through the intertragic notch as if it were a small window. Then place your probe within it and feel for the deepest depression; that is the point.	This point assists in regulating water passageways. It connects all three *Jiaos*. By doing so, it can be used to eliminate excess water or Damp. It facilitates digestion and distributes the Essential Substances to the entire body. It strengthens immunity and can be used to fight off exogenous evils. It can be used for constipation and edema.
#48 Duodenum	Cymba Concha	In the 1st sector.	This point is for problems of the duodenum, such as duodenal ulcer. It assists in the absorptive aspects of digestion.

(*continued*)

Table 4.1 (continued). Auricular Acupuncture Points: Location and Energetics

Point	Ear Zone	Specific Location	Energetics
#49 Small Intestine	Cymba Concha	In the 2nd sector.	This point can be used for problems of the Small Intestine, such as digestive disturbances, particularly absorption problems. It aids in the separation of the pure from the impure. Also used for palpitations due to its connection to the Heart.
#50 Large Intestine	Cymba Concha	In the 3rd sector.	The Large Intestine point can regulate the Large Intestine in any condition. It helps with water absorption, ulcerative colitis, loose stools and/or constipation, hemorrhoids, irritable bowel syndrome, and other Large Intestine maladies.
#51 Appendix	Cymba Concha	At the junction of the 2nd and 3rd sectors (between the Small Intestine and the Large Intestine points).	This point is for inflammation of the vermiform appendix (acute simple appendicitis).
#52 Bladder	Cymba Concha	In the 4th sector, directly above the Large Intestine point.	The Bladder point is for problems, such as urinary incontinence, frequency of urination, enuresis, retention of urine, dribbling urination, urinary urgency, difficult urination, painful urination, stones, bladder infections, cloudy urination, and other urinary problems.

#53 Kidney	Cymba Concha	In the 5th sector, directly above the Small Intestine point.	The Kidney point can be utilized for a vast array of disorders that are subsumed under "Kidney" in Oriental medicine. Such disorders include problems connected with Bladder function, foundation *Yin* and *Yang*, problems of growth, maturation, and development. It treats immune disorders, builds blood, and regulates body warmth. It can be used for kidney stones, nephritis, lumbago, tinnitus, and other Kidney problems.
#54 Ureters	Cymba Concha	At the junction of the 4th and 5th sectors (between the Kidney and Bladder points).	This point is used for stones that may collect in the ureters or to assist in the elimination of urine.
#55 Pancreas/ Gallbladder	Cymba Concha	In the 6th sector, directly above the Duodenum point.	This area assists in sugar/insulin regulation, and promotes proper bile regulation. It assists in the breakdown of fats and helps the Liver in its *Yang* functional aspects. It treats cholecystitis, cholelithiasis, gallstones, and other problems of the Gallbladder and Pancreas. Dr. So (1987, p. 48) and Nogier claim that the Pancreas point is treated in the left ear and the Gall Bladder point in the right. For pancreatitis and diseases of the bile duct.

(*continued*)

Table 4.1 (continued). Auricular Acupuncture Points: Location and Energetics

Point	Ear Zone	Specific Location	Energetics
#56 Diaphragm	Helix	Near the lateral edge on the crus of the helix.	The Diaphragm is a powerful point for moving the diaphragm, thus assisting in deep breathing. When the diaphragm moves, Liver *Qi* is regulated and the distribution of *Qi* and Blood in the upper *Jiao* is facilitated. It is a major point for the treatment of *Qi* and Blood Stagnation. It has an effect upon the emotions by virtue of moving Liver *Qi* stagnation. For hiccup and jaundice. It helps the Upper *Jiao* and the Middle *Jiao* communicate better and dispels chest and midback tightness. Some authors refer to this point as Point Zero or the Master point. Because it corresponds to the diaphragm, it is good for nervous tension, hiccups, and pressure from the Stomach or Liver following surgery. It has mixed sympathetic/parasympathetic innervations. Kropej recommends needling it first in a treatment because it affects the reactive ability of the rest of the auricle. It can make an unreactive or a hypersensitive ear normalized.
#57 Lower Portion of the Rectum	Helix	On the helix, roughly parallel to the Large Intestine point.	This point is for problems, such as fecal stagnation, constipation, impacted stools, hemorrhoids, diverticulitis, and diverticuloses of the lower rectum.
#58 Hemorrhoids	Helix	On the border of the helix, parallel to the Uterus/ Prostate	This is a point specifically for hemorrhoids due to Stagnant Blood, Damp-Heat accumulation or prolapsed *Qi*. Also treats itchiness, inflammation, bleeding, and anal fissures.

#59 Common Cold	Helix	On the border of the helix, parallel to the Hypertension point.	This point can be used to help prevent the common cold or to treat it if already developed. It can be used for symptoms of Wind-Cold, Heat, or Dampness that cause common cold manifestations.
#60 Ear Apex	Helix	**Tip:** At the top of the helix, this point is found by folding the helix gently. The point is at the top of the fold.	This is an important point to bring down *Yang* and reduce Heat. In the case of subduing *Yang*, this point reduces high blood pressure and can quell anger and the heat manifestations of *Yang* Rising. It is a clinically effective point for conjunctivitis, migraines, and other symptoms of Liver *Yang* Rising.
#61 Helix 1 #62 Helix 2 #63 Helix 3 #64 Helix 4	Helix Helix Helix Helix	Found by dividing the helix into six equal parts respectively. The first point is on the helix, parallel to the tubercle of the helix and the sixth point is found in sector 8 of the lobe. All others are found in between those divisions at equal intervals. Helix 5 and 6 have already been numbered as points 17 and 19.	These points pertain to tonsillar tissue and can be used to enhance immunity and ward off infection or invasion. For acute tonsillitis.

(*continued*)

Table 4.1 (continued). Auricular Acupuncture Points: Location and Energetics

Point	Ear Zone	Specific Location	Energetics
#65 *Dingchuan*	Antitragus	At the height or the apex of the antitragus (not on the anterior surface, but exactly on the top of it).	This is another very powerful point to assist in stop wheezing, analogous to *Dingchuan* on the back of the neck (0.5 cun lateral to DU 14). It is excellent for bronchitis, asthma, and other disorders where there are breathing difficulties and wheezing. It works well with the *Stop Wheezing* point in the triangular fossa.
#66 Brain	Antitragus	On the posterior wall of the antitragus.	The Brain point is involved in regulating the excitation and inhibition of the cerebral cortex. It is for diseases of the nervous, digestive, endocrine, and urogenital systems, hemorrhage, insomnia, inflammation, pain, swelling, shock, prolapse, and excessive sweating. To me, it is the second most important point to *Shenmen* and can be used to augment virtually every treatment because the brain controls all bodily activity.
#67 Occiput	Antitragus	The most lateral of the three points.	The Occiput is a local point for the occipital area, such as in the case of occipital headaches, neck tension, stiffness along the nape, and Blood Stasis patterns in the occipital area. Additionally, it pertains to the occipital lobe, which is where the visual cortex of the brain is located, so this point can be used for multiple eye disorders. It treats neuropsychiatric disorders, psychosis, pain, shock, inflammation, convulsions, lockjaw, and nervous system regulation. It can also be used for motion sickness, dizziness, and headache.

#68 Temple, also called *Taiyang*	Antitragus	Midway between Occiput and Temple.	This is a local point for problems of the temple, such as breakouts, tension, etc. It is good for temporal headaches, one-sided headaches, and migraines.
#69 Forehead	Antitragus	The most medial of these three points.	This local point is for problems of the forehead, such as wrinkles, acne, pain and congestion of the sinuses and forehead. It is used to treat *Yangming* Stomach/Large Intestine headaches.
#70 Brainstem	Antitragus	Just above the antitragus area. It is created by the intersection of the medial border of the Spleen and the area above the antitragus.	This point is for disorders of the cerebral blood vessels and meninges, incomplete development of the brain, apoplexy, convulsions, stiffness along the nape, sequel to cerebral shock, primitive brain function, and respiration.
#71 Eye 1	Antitragus	On the medial side of the intertragic notch.	These are supplemental points for a wide array of eye disorders. Use with the Eye point on the lobe as the primary point. For glaucoma and myopia.
#72 Eye 2	Antitragus	On the lateral side of the intertragic notch.	
#73 Raise Blood Pressure	Antitragus	Below the intertragic notch between Eye 1 and Eye 2.	This useful point can treat low blood pressure. It is an emergency point to raise blood pressure.
#74 Ovaries/Testes	Antitragus	Slightly superior to Eye 2.	In both men and women, this point can be used to treat a variety of reproductive disorders involving the ovaries or the testes. For irregular menstruation and epididymitis.

#75 Endocrine	Antitragus	On the medial side of the intertragic notch, superior to Eye 1, on the posterior wall of the medial border of the intertragic notch.	This point is used to regulate all endocrine secretions in the body; thus, it is used for hormonal problems.
#76 Toe	Superior Antihelix Crus	Toe is the most lateral point, found where the inverted L begins.	This point can be used for diverse toe problems, such as fractures, bunions, hammer toes, arthritis, and other traumatic disorders.
#77 Heel	Superior Antihelix Crus	Heel is in between, at the junction of the two strokes that form the L.	This point can be used for heel problems, such as calcaneal spurs.
#78 Ankle	Superior Antihelix Crus	Ankle is inferior to the heel at the point where the L ends.	This point is for ankle problems, such as breaks, sprains, swelling, and other ankle problems.
#79 Knee	Superior Antihelix Crus	This is an area found superior to where the superior antihelix crus intersects with the inferior antihelix crus.	For a variety of knee problems, such as knee crepitation, achiness, cold knees, disorders involving ligaments or the joint, or for knee circulation problems.
#80 Lumbago	Antihelix	Found exactly at the intersection of the superior and inferior antihelix crura.	This is an excellent clinically effective point for low back pain in the lumbar region.
#81 Sciatic Nerve	Inferior Antihelix Crus	In the center of the inferior antihelix crus at its most medial location.	Another quick acting, clinically effective point for the clinical manifestations of a compressed sciatic nerve causing radiating pain down the side or the back of the leg.

#82 Ischium	Inferior Antihelix Crus	Just below the triangular fossa, in the inferior antihelix crus, slightly medial to the Buttocks point.	The Ischium point is for problems originating out of the buttocks, such as sciatica or problems pertaining to the ischium, the lower portion of the hipbone.
#83 Buttocks	Inferior Antihelix Crus	Just below the triangular fossa, in the inferior antihelix crus, slightly lateral to Ischium.	Buttocks can be used similarly as the Ischium point or for other gluteal problems.
#84 Abdomen	Antihelix	Area on the lower antihelix crus roughly parallel to the Liver and Pancreas/Gallbladder points.	The Abdomen point is good for general, diffuse, or specific abdominal problems. It can be treated alone or in combination with a specific part of the abdomen, such as the Large Intestine, Appendix, etc.
#85 Chest	Antihelix	Area in the lower antihelix crus roughly parallel to the Stomach point.	This point can be used for a vast array of chest problems, such as tightness in the chest, shortness of breath, asthma, cough, cold, and other respiratory or chest disorders. Like the Abdomen it can be used singularly or in combination with other points that are in this region, such as the Mammary points, Lung, Heart, etc.
#86, 87 Mammary Glands	Antihelix	Below the chest area, roughly parallel to the center of the Spleen. There are two of them positioned next to each other.	These are two excellent clinically effective points for the treatment of fibrocystic breast disease, breast distention, and tenderness.

(*continued*)

Table 4.1 (continued). Auricular Acupuncture Points: Location and Energetics

Point	Ear Zone	Specific Location	Energetics
#88 Neck	Antihelix	On the lower antihelix crus, roughly parallel to the curvature of the antihelix, above the antitragus.	The Neck is a fast-working point for a host of neck problems, such as stiff neck, torticollis, and misaligned vertebrae.
#89 Throat and Teeth	Antihelix	Below the Neck, slightly above the Occiput point.	These points are for throat problems, such as tonsillitis, sore throat, and constriction in the throat as well as a general point for teeth problems.
#90 Sacral Vertebrae	Antihelix	Extends from the most medial portion of the inferior antihelix crus to about parallel to the end of the Bladder point.	Each pertains to a particular segment of the spinal column. They are superb points to use when these portions of the spinal cord are involved. They are especially effective for adjusting the vertebrae. Additionally they can be used for treating the nerves that originate from particular portions of the spinal cord and the organs, areas, and dermatomes that they innervate.
#91 Lumbar Vertebrae	Antihelix	From the end of the sacral area, parallel to about the middle of the Liver area.	
#92 Thoracic Vertebrae	Antihelix	Extends from the end of the Lumbar area to just above the curvature of the lower antihelix crus.	

#93 Cervical Vertebrae	Antihelix	Extends from the end of the Thoracic area to the end of the curvature of the lower antihelix.	
#94 Vagus Root, also called Ear Root or Root of the Auricular Vagus Nerve	Posterior Aspect	In the depression just above the ear root (where the ear attaches to the head, above the tendon). **Tip:** To locate, pull the ear laterally. This will isolate the tendon to assist in locating the point. The point is in the depression above the tendon.	This is a powerful point to regulate functions of the Middle *Jiao*. It is used for digestive disorders, gastralgia, and helps to expel gallstones. It is also for headaches, asthma, stomachache, palpitations, bowel problems, and all areas that the vagus nerve, the longest cranial nerve in the body, innervates.
#95 Upper Back #96 Middle Back #97 Lower Back	Posterior Aspect Posterior Aspect Posterior Aspect	Along the spiny cartilaginous middle portion of the back of the ear, respectively. According to *Chinese Acupuncture and Moxibustion*, the Upper Back is on top, the Middle is in the middle, and the Lower Back is on the bottom.	These local points correspond to a variety of back problems. It is helpful to use these with the corresponding type of back pain points on the front of the ear for added reinforcement. For instance, use Upper Back with Upper Thoracic.

(continued)

Table 4.1 (continued). Auricular Acupuncture Points: Location and Energetics

Point	Ear Zone	Specific Location	Energetics
#98 Lower Blood Pressure Groove	Posterior Aspect	A groove-like depression on the posterior aspect of the ear formed by the posterior border of the helix. It runs approximately the length of the upper third of the groove.	This is a very powerful area to lower high blood pressure when bled (to be discussed under modalities, Chapter 6).
#99 Superior Root of Ear	Posterior Aspect	On the posterior aspect of the ear at the intersection of the superior part of the auricle with the face.	This point treats hemiplegia.
#100 Spinal Cord 1	Posterior Aspect	On the posterior aspect of the ear, at the superior border of the inferior annicular root.	This point can be used for muscular atrophy and paralysis.

References

1. Richards, D. and Marley, J. Stimulation of auricular points in weight loss. *Aus. Fam. Phys.*, 1998, July 27 (Suppl.) 2: 73–77.
2. Helms, J. *Acupuncture Energetics: A Clinical Approach for Physicians.* Medical Acupuncture Publishers, Berkeley, CA, 1995, p. 136.
3. Romoli, M. and Giomi, A. Ear acupuncture in psychosomatic medicine: the importance of the *Sanjiao* (triple heater) area. *Acpunc. Electrother. Res.*, 1993, Jul.–Dec., 18(3–4): 185–194.
4. So, J. *Treatment of Disease with Acupuncture.* Paradigm Publications, Brookline, MA, 1987, p. 50.
5. Kropej, H. *The Fundamental of Ear Acupuncture,* 4th ed. Karl F. Haug Publishers, Heidelberg, Germany, 1991, p. 31.
6. Soliman, N.E. and Frank, B.L. *Atlas of Auricular Therapy and Auricular Medicine.* Integrated Medicine Publishers, Richardson, TX, 1999, p. 62.
7. Nanking Army Ear Acupuncture Team. Huang, H. (trans.). *Ear Acupuncture.* Rodale Press, Emmanus, PA, 1974, p. 79.

Bibliography

Ciu, Y. Needling auricular point Heart in treatment of dysphonia: report of 170 cases. *Int. J. Clin. Acupunc.*, 1993, 4(3): 273–276.

Dai, J. and Liang, S. A clinical observation on coronary heart disease treated at heart otopoint. *J. Trad. Chin. Med.*, 1998, 18(1): 43–46.

Goa, J., Shi, X., Wang, J., Zhu, B., Hu, Z., Yu, M., Zhong, Y., and Xing, J. Recognition of multiple information of human auricular points by linear model. *Sheng Wu Yi Xue Gong Cheng Xue Za Zhi*, 2000 Sept., 17(3): 316–319, (in Chinese).

Gong, C.M. Observation with real-time ultrasound on GB contraceptive effects with-EAP of earpoint GB. *Am. J. Acupunc.*, 1988, 16: 181.

He, T. Treatment of acute lumbar sprain with otoacupuncture at the acupoint lumbago. *J. Trad. Chin. Med.*, June 1993, 13(2): 106.

Helms, J. *Acupuncture Energetics: A Clinical Approach for Physicians.* Medical Acupuncture Publishers, Berkeley, CA, 1995.

Hep, A., Prasek, J., Dolina, J., Ondrousek, L., and Dite, P. Treatment of esophageal motility disorders with acupuncture of the ear. *Vnitr. Lek.*, 1995 July, 41(7): 473–475, (in Czech).

Huang, H. et al. Acupuncture at otopoint heart for treatment of vascular hypertension. *J. Trad. Chin. Med.*, June 1992, 12(2): 133–136.

Jian, L.X. Therapeutic effects of auricular acupoints in ear acupuncture. *Heilongjiang Trad. Chin. Med. Mater. Med.*, 1990, 3: 42–43.

Kropej, H. *The Fundamental of Ear Acupuncture,* 4th ed. Karl F. Haug Publishers, Heidelberg, Germany, 1991.

Liu, W. and Xu, G. An approach to mechanism of function of auricular point. *Zhen Ci* Yan *Jiu*, 1990, 15(3): 187–190, (in Chinese).

Liu, W.Z., Yang, Y.B., and Li, D.Z. Observation of the relative specificity between the stimulated auricular point and propagated sensation along channel (PSC). *Zhen Ci Yan Jiu*, 1986, 11(2): 158–161, (in Chinese).

Nanking Army Ear Acupuncture Team. Huang, H. (trans.). *Ear Acupuncture.* Rodale Press, Emmanus, PA, 1974, p. 79.

Oleson, T. and Kroening, R. A new nomenclature for identifying Chinese and Nogier auricular acupuncture points. *Am. J. Acupunc.*, Oct.–Dec. 1983, 11(4).

Oleson, T. and Kroening, R. A comparison of Chinese and Nogier auricular acupuncture points. *Am. J. Acupunc.*, Jul.–Sept. 1983, 11(3): 205–223.

Richards, D. and Marley, J. Stimulation of auricular points in weight loss. *Aus. Fam. Phys.*, 1998 Jul. 27, (Suppl.) 2: 73–77.

Romoli, M. and Giomi, A. Ear acupuncture in psychosomatic medicine: the importance of the *Sanjiao* (triple heater) area. *Acupunc. Electrother. Res.*, 1993, Jul.–Dec., 18(3–4): 185–194.

So, J. *Treatment of Disease with Acupuncture.* Paradigm Publications, Brookline, MA, 1987.

Soliman, N.E. and Frank, B.L. *Atlas of Auricular Therapy and Auricular Medicine.* Integrated Medicine Publishers, Richardson, TX, 1999.

chapter five

Cautions and contraindications

Objective

- To review conditions under which ear acupuncture is either contraindicated or where caution should be used to prevent harm to the patient

Introduction

As discussed in Chapter 4, the ear points, like the body acupuncture points, have a broad range of clinical application. Both can be used for the diagnosis, treatment, and prevention of human health disorders. However, according to clinical experience and classical theory, as with body acupuncture points, there are certain conditions under which ear acupuncture is either contraindicated or when caution should be used so that no harm is done to the patient.

Due to these possible serious complications, conditions of contraindication and caution are discussed first, prior to the ear modalities covered in Chapter 6. Thus, these potential dangers can be foremost in the practitioner's mind in preparation for treatment.

Pregnancy

In my opinion and that of many other practitioners, auricular acupuncture on a pregnant woman is absolutely forbidden. Because of the strong manner in which the ear moves *Qi* and Blood, an unwanted miscarriage could ensue from the use of ear acupuncture. The ear can be used to promote the health of the woman who wishes to become pregnant and to help her recover after delivery, but it is very risky to use during the gestation period. As a result I do not treat pregnant women with ear modalities, but there are those who disagree with this contraindication.

Skin problems

Avoid applying ear modalities to rashes, moles, scars, skin reconstructed through plastic surgery, irritated ear skin, frostbitten skin, ear abrasions, or other skin breakouts in the ear. Treating unhealed skin on the ear can lead to further irritation, pain, and infection. Wait until the ear heals before treating with auricular modalities. Do not needle into unidentifiable lumps or lesions. Refer the patient to a dermatologist if you are suspicious of any observed anomaly.

Special considerations

Weak patients, immunocompromised patients, children, patients with bleeding disorders and tumors

Use ear acupuncture with caution on patients who have poor wound-healing capacity, such as immunocompromised patients who are prone to infection. Cancer patients, diabetics, those who have HIV positive status, or others with immune disorders fall into this category. Use ear acupuncture prudently on hemophiliacs, diabetic patients, the elderly, and others who tend to bleed easily; those with impaired neurological functioning or patients on pain medications who may not detect pain or *Qi* arrival.

> ***Note:*** Patients with high blood pressure may bleed more easily than others. You can still use ear-bleeding techniques on these patients. In fact, bleeding is the preferred modality for certain varieties of hypertension characterized by excess Heat and *Yang Rising*. Be prepared for possible bleeding. Wear gloves and have extra cotton balls nearby.

Do not use ear acupuncture on young children who might remove ear seeds or pellets and put them into his or her mouth or nose. Except for life-threatening circumstances, do not use ear acupuncture on children under the age of seven, so as not to disturb the body's developmental processes. Ear massage administered by a professional or by a parent instructed in how to perform such massage is a good alternative to pellets and seeds.

Use auricular therapy with caution on weakened patients, elderly patients, or patients with decreased functional mental ability. Patients with severe psychological problems may not respond properly to the signs of *Qi* arrival or be able to follow instructions even if the instructions are written down. Written directions are always a good idea for properly informing the patient of instructions and advice.

Use caution with ear modalities applied close to the external auditory meatus so that they do not fall into the ear canal. Several such written directions pertaining to auricular acupuncture are found in Chapter 6 on the ear modalities.

Due to the possibility of metastasis, do not use ear acupuncture on cancer patients. However, the ear is an excellent modality for treating cancer patients after the tumor has been removed and during chemotherapy and/or radiation treatment to assist in promoting well-being, strengthening organ function, and rebuilding immunity.

Pain and other variables

One of the chief indications for auriculoacupuncture is the remediation of pain. If the underlying etiology of that pain is not addressed with Oriental or Western therapeutics, pain relief may only be temporary and even dangerous.

Noted auricular acupuncturist Paul Nogier provides a list of other disorders for which he claims ear acupuncture is contraindicated. He warns not to use for "neuroleptics; if there is vertebral blockage as in the case of disc herniation; for paralysis; and if the patient has a permanent scar condition."[1]

Likewise, Helmut Kropej has a set of what he calls absolute contraindications for ear therapy. He cautions not to use ear acupuncture for the following conditions: "Pain that necessitates surgery, demyelinating diseases, treatment of the thalamus and inner genitals during pregnancy, and all congenital disorders in which the spinal cord is mainly affected." He furthers maintains that hormonally active points during menstruation should not be used.[2] I have not found the latter to be a problem.

Side effects

Occasionally, following ear acupuncture treatment, the ear may develop an adverse skin reaction. Every precaution must be taken to avert any skin inflammation as a result of the ear treatment. Thorough asepsis of the ear by means of clean needle technique must be maintained to prevent infection to the delicate auricle. All treatment materials positioned in the ear must be sterile. Remember that the ear is richly supplied with lymphatic vessels, thus making the ear particularly susceptible to infection.

Infection of the ear, known as auricular perichondritis, has been the subject of many studies. O. Davis states, "Acupuncture must be considered a form of penetrating trauma that may induce a perichondritis or chondritis in the auricle."[3] In one such study, Johansen and Nielson wrote, "Repeated cultures showed growth of *Pseudomonas aeruginosa*. Despite intensive antibiotic treatment and extensive surgical toilet, the patient developed a severely deformed outer ear."[4] Of particular danger is penetration of the perichondrium by needles, tacks, and intradermals.

Palle Rosted shows that "the inoculation of organisms into the subperichondral plane can occur. The chronic presence of a foreign body further impairs the host's ability to eradicate infection. Permanent cosmetic changes to the ear may ensue. Repeated manipulation of implanted needles can cause further irritation and subperichondrial inoculation. This can happen to all patients, especially those who have diabetes, are immunosuppressed, or have a chronic debilitating disease."[5]

Retention of the ear treatment modality for too long or under improper conditions may be precipitating factors in ear infection. The metal the modality is composed of is also correlated with skin reactions. Rosted notes that "skin reactions in the form of eczema may develop in patients sensitive to nickel, chromium, or silver. Stainless steel has been known to produce free nickel in certain situations."[5] F. Leggat et al. claim that "small particles of silver from a needle may accidentally be deposited in the ear, leading to the development of localized cutaneous argyria presenting as a blue-black macule in the skin."[6]

As with all acupuncture treatment, there are certain conditions under which ear acupuncture should not be administered, as it can create undesirable side effects. These contraindications include:

- A patient who is overtired, physically or mentally. Treatment at this time can further weaken the patient and the *Qi* that is already in a deficient state. Light-headedness or fainting can result.
- A patient who is under the influence of mind-altering drugs, including alcohol; treatment should be postponed.
- A patient who has overeaten; he/she may be uncomfortable or unresponsive during treatment. Conversely, if the patient is very hungry (considered a weakened state), acupuncture also should be postponed.

The potential signs of acupuncture-induced illness in auricular acupuncture are the same as with body acupuncture. They include dizziness, palpitations, cold sweats, nausea, chest tightness, fidgeting, weak pulse, fainting, and even unconsciousness.

Positioning of patients

Ear acupuncture can be administered in a sitting or a reclining position. I follow these general guidelines.

- If the ear is to be needled or bled, I have the patient lie down, as the manipulation of *Qi* and Blood can make the patient feel weak or faint.
- If more gentle modalities, such as pellets or seeds, are part of the "take-home" treatment, the therapy may be applied while the patient is sitting or reclining. The position depends upon what is comfortable to the patient or where the practitioner is in the treatment when the seeds are applied (i.e., at the beginning or the end of treatment).

The conditions for successful treatment of the patient can be achieved by proper positioning of patients as well as adherence to the prohibitions listed above.

References

1. Nogier, P. *Handbook of Auriculotherapy.* Maisonneuve, Moulins-les–Metz, France, 1981, p. 121.
2. Kropej, H. *The Fundamentals of Ear Acupuncture, 4th ed.* Karl F. Haug Publishers, Heidelberg, Germany; 1991, p. 27.
3. Davis, O. and Powell, W. Auricular perichondritis secondary to acupuncture. *Arch. Otolaryngol.*, 1985 Nov., 111(11): 770–771.
4. Johansen, M. and Nielson, K.O. Perichondritis of the ear canal caused by acupuncture. *Ugeskr. Laeger.*, 1990 Jan. 15, 152(3): 172–173, (in Danish).
5. Rosted, P. Adverse reactions after acupuncture: a review. *Am. J. Acupunc.*, 1996, 24: 27–34.
6. Legart, F.J., Goessler, W., Schlagenhaufen, C., and Soyer, H.P. Localized cutaneous argyria in the ear after short-contact acupuncture. *Acta Dermt. Venereol.*, 1999, 8(4): 89, (in Norwegian).

Bibliography

Allison, G. and Kravitz, E. Auricular chondritis secondary to acupuncture. *New Eng. J. Med.*, 1975, 273: 780.

Alter, M.J. Hepatitis C virus infection in the United States. *J. Hepatol.*, 1999, 31 (Suppl.) 1: 88–91.

Baltimore, R.S. and Moloy, P.J. Perichondritis of the ear as a complication of acupuncture. *Arch. Otolaryngol.*, 1976, 102: 572–573.

Bork, K. Multiple lymphocytoma at the point of puncture as complication of acupuncture treatment: traumatic origin of lymphocytoma. *Hautarzt.*, 1983, Oct., 34(10): 496–499, (in German).

Dahlquist, A. and Johnsen, J. A warning against ear acupuncture used in the treatment of obesity. *Lakartidningen*, 1987, Sept. 16, 84(38): 2970, (in Swedish).

Davis, O. and Powell, W. Auricular perichondritis secondary to acupuncture. *Arch. Otolaryngol.*, 1985, Nov., 111(11): 770–771.

Gilbert, J.G. Auricular complication of acupuncture. *N.Z. Med. J.*, 1987, Mar. 112, 100(819): 141–142.

Johansen, M. and Nielson, K.O. Perichondritis auriculae forarsaget af akupunkturbehandling. *Ugeskr. Laeger.*, 1990, 152(3): 172, (in Danish).

Jones, H.S. Auricular complications of acupuncture. *J. Laryngol. Otol.*, 1985, 99: 1143–1145.

Kropej, H. *The Fundamentals of Ear Acupuncture, 4th ed.*. Karl F. Haug Publishers, Heidelberg, Germany; 1991.

Lee, R.J. and Mc Ilwain, J.C. Subacute bacterial endocarditis following ear acupuncture. *Int. J. Cardiol.*, 1985 Jan., 7(1): 62–63.

Legart, F.J., Goessler, W., Schlagenhaufen, C., and Soyer, H.P. Localized cutaneous argyria in the ear after short-contact acupuncture. *Acta Dermtol. Venereol.*, 1999, 8(4): 89, (in Norwegian).

Nogier, P. *Handbook of Auriculotherapy.* Maisonneuve, Moulins-les–Metz, France, 1981.

Peacher, W.G. Adverse reactions, contraindications, and complications of acupuncture and moxibustion. *Am. J. Chin. Med.*, 1975 Jan., 3(1): 35–46.

Rosted, P. Adverse reactions after acupuncture: a review. *Am. J. Acupunc.*, 1996, 24: 27–34.

Savage, J.H. Auricular complications of acupuncture. *J. Laryngol. Otol.*, 1985 Nov., 99(11): 1143–1145.

Sorenson, T. Auricular perichondritis caused by acupuncture therapy. *Ugeskr. Laefer.*, 1990 Mar. 12, 152(11): 752–753, (in Danish).

Tang, C. Treatment of adverse reactions following facial cosmetic surgical abrasion with auricular pellet therapy. *J. Trad. Chin. Med.*, 1990 Sept., 10(3): 196–198.

Wedenberg, K., Moer, B., and Norling, A. A prospective randomized study comparing acupuncture with physiotherapy for low-back and pelvic pain in pregnancy. *Acta Obstet. Gynecol. Scand.*, 2000, 79(5): 331–335, (in Scandinavian).

chapter six

Ear modalities

Objectives

- To explore 15 of the most common modalities used in auricular medicine
- To gain an understanding of which side of the ear to treat
- To understand the expected therapeutic results of treatment

Introduction

Auricular acupuncture may be chosen either as a primary treatment method or as a complementary adjunct to address a patient's illness. Whether for the management of an acute emergency, for treatment of initial symptoms or chronic problems, or for preventative treatment, there is a wide range of modalities that an acupuncturist can use. Although some of these modalities are similar in nature (such as seeds, tacks, and pellets), each has some unique feature. As a practitioner, you have the option of selecting a modality from a number of criteria, such as those modalities that have the highest degree of clinical efficacy for the condition to be treated, the modality that best meets the lifestyle and compliance level of the patient, as well as modalities that satisfy your comfort level or preference as a practitioner. Ear modalities include:

- Palpation and massage
- Needles
- Ear seeds and herbal plasters
- Pellets
- Tacks
- Intradermal needles
- Magnets
- Electroacupuncture
- Bleeding
- Moxibustion

- Incisions/sutures
- Injections
- Lasers
- Staples
- Plum blossom needling

Certain ear points and particular ear acupuncture modalities are clinically correlated with some specific medical conditions. Where relevant, such conditions are discussed in relation to the modalities so as to convey to the reader the most precise use of those points and treatment options.

Keep in mind that regardless of the modality selected, strict asepsis of the ear must be maintained to prevent infection from developing. Use a hair clip to secure the patient's hair away from the ear so that it does not contaminate the auricle during treatment or become attached to the sticky tapes of the pellets, magnets, and seeds. Remove ear jewelry, piercings, or hearing aids for massage, diagnosis, or other modalities as needed. Table 6.1 summarizes the use of the ear modalities (numbered 1 to 15) discussed in this chapter.

Palpation and massage (1)

Palpation is the process of detecting tender points for diagnosis or treatment by pressing on the ear point. These same points can be treated by rubbing or applying pressure to the point.

A healthy ear point, like a healthy body acupuncture point, should not be tender when pressed or palpated. Tenderness through pressure indicates a problem in the area being tested. Paul Nogier accurately points out that "this does not mean that all pathology is reflected in the ear as it may take time for that pathology to be conveyed to the site. Additionally, this is more likely if there are problems with nervous transmission of information."[1]

To perform palpation, use a sterile, stainless steel ear probe (Figure 6.1). Although the probe does not pierce the skin, there is still the possibility of spreading infection from person to person via an unsterilized probe. Therefore, ear probes should be sterile for each patient. Do not swab the ear with alcohol prior to palpation as the alcohol may change the skin's electrical conductivity or remove pathological discharges, such as suppurations, thus affecting the clinical data derived from observation or palpation.

From an Oriental perspective, when performing ear diagnosis, it is not advisable or necessary to palpate every ear point. First, establish the working diagnosis. Pathology observed in the ear, along with data from other methods, can be used to substantiate a diagnosis. Points relating to the diagnosis can be then palpated and the sensitivity of the ear, if any, used as supporting data.

Apply equal pressure in palpating the points you consider using in your prescription. Points for treatment may be marked by pressing with the probe, or by using a sterile, gentian violet marking pen, or simply by remembering the points. After palpation, such points are generally treated with an ear modality or even with the probe employed as a massage device.

Table 6.1 Auricular Modalities

Modalities	Conditions
1. Palpation and Massage	Massage can be applied by the therapist or the patient after the patient is instructed on where and how to massage the ear. Mark the spot to be massaged with a pellet or sterile marking pen.
2. Needles	Needling is the most common auricular therapeutic modality. Needles can be inserted into any point. Insert — get *Qi* — then tonify or disperse. Heat is the most desired stimulus of *Qi* arrival. *Note:* I tend not to needle the Heart, Brain, *Dingchuan*, Vagus, or points on the lobe unless needed because of their strong effect. For these points, I substitute pellets. However, they are not contraindicated to needle.
3. Ear Seeds and Herbal Plasters	Seeds provide a good stimulus due to their size and density. However, if they are not sterile, they can increase the risk of infection. Herbal deposits on the seeds can impart herbal therapeutic benefits.
4. Ear Pellets: gold, silver, or other metals	Pellets are a good size modality for auricular treatment. They provide a perfect stimulus and have the added benefit of being sterile. Additionally, pellets are available in various metals. Therefore, pellets can also be used for their metallurgic properties.
5. Ear Tacks	Tacks come in various sizes — extra small, small, medium, and large. The bigger the tac, the stronger the stimulus, so consider patient tolerance when choosing the tack size. There can be a higher risk of infection with ear tacks if patients do not have the tacks removed at the proper time.
6. Intradermal Needles	Intradermal needles are used for areas such as the Constipation or Vertebral areas. Do not use in depressions. The intradermal needle will not go into a depression easily and may break. Intradermal needles need to be placed on points on a ridge or flat area. Intradermals are available in various lengths. Select the appropriate length based on the size of the point to be needled.
7. Magnets	Magnets need to be removed at bedtime or if the stimulus becomes too strong for the patient. They are reusable on the same patient. Magnets do not pierce the skin, thus the risk of infection is reduced.
8. Electroacupuncture	Electricity is good for anaesthetizing a point due to the electrical machine's ability to achieve high frequencies that stimulate the point. Do not clean the ear with alcohol prior to using the point detector for diagnosis, as this will change the ear pathology and the electrical resistance of the ear.

(*continued*)

Table 6.1 (continued) Auricular Modalities

Modalities	Conditions
9. Bleeding	Bleeding is used to reduce Heat/Fire, subdue *Yang*, stimulate *Qi* and Blood, or to move Stagnant *Qi* and Blood.
10. Moxibustion	Moxa use is limited, but specific to treating earache or the common cold and other conditions. It can be applied indirectly over the point or over a needle.
11. Incisions/Sutures	Incisions/sutures are a technique that is typically not employed in the U.S. because an incision is considered a surgical technique. An incision provides a constant stimulus to the point. Chances of infection are increased using incisions.
12. Injections	Injections can be applied to the point with a hypodermic needle. Common injections include saline, vitamin B_{12}, certain Chinese herbal formulations, lidocaine, procaine, and placenta. This procedure is slightly painful due to the small size of the point, the size of the hypodermic needle, and the nature of the substance injected.
13. Laser	Laser therapy is one of the newest modalities. It is painless and infection is not an issue. Ease of administration also makes it a good choice in treatment.
14. Staples	Like incisions and sutures, this is an old technique used to stimulate points. Seeds or pellets are commonly used now in the place of staples.
15. Plum Blossom Needling	This modality may be applied to points of the lobe as well as used as a method to induce bleeding in the ear.

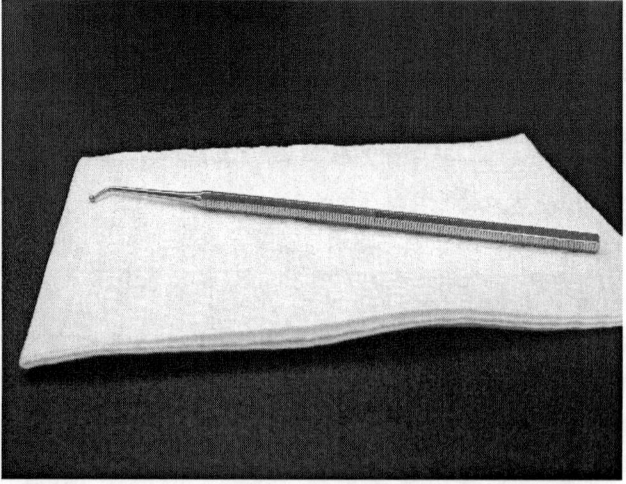

Figure 6.1 Ear probe.

Massage

Just as palpation is used for diagnosis, palpation is also used as a massage technique by either the patient through self-treatment or by a practitioner. Ear massage is a relaxing, enjoyable, noninvasive, and clinically effective modality for the treatment of most health disorders. Massage can encompass the entire auricle or it can focus on specific treatment points. I recommend doing both.

Chinese folk culture abounds in tales of "pulling" on the ears 300 times every day to ensure a healthy life and promote longevity. Many Chinese have a story about a relative or friend who lived into his or her one hundreds because that relative or friend practiced ear massage regularly. A Qing dynasty text reads, "Massaging the helix with the hands for a number of times is also called reinforcing the city wall to tonify the Kidney *Qi*, prevent deafness, and treat insomnia."[2]

The Chinese maintain that the ears, which pertain to the Kidney, are the direct manifestation of "fortune" – what the Chinese construe as health, wealth, longevity, and prosperity. The Chinese say, "The bigger the ear, the bigger the fortune." Other cultures have also viewed the ear as indicative of stamina, status, a sign of Buddhahood, or even representing the seat of the soul."[3]

While practitioners have their preferences, there are no set ways to massage the ear. My massage method is more of an "even" technique that disperses tension and, yet, simultaneously brings energy to (tonifies) areas of deficiency. Keep the massage simple and short. An overly complex method will be difficult for the patient or practitioner to follow and execute. Massaging the ear for too long will tend to disperse the patient's energy.

The patient should remain silent during this treatment so that his energy is allowed to go deep into his body. If you want, you can lead the patient through a guided visualization of what you are doing and how the points correlate with the specific body parts so the patient can develop awareness about the points. However, because this is a treatment that requires quietude, avoid discussion. By treating the whole ear, all of the points are stimulated, thereby treating the person in a very comprehensive way. Preferably, overall ear massage should be done prior to the body acupuncture treatment. Massage at the end of the treatment disrupts the focus achieved through the body acupuncture. Patients love ear massage. It takes only a few minutes to administer and, based on my own clinical experience and patient feedback, has a positive effect on balancing body energetics.

Ear massage protocol

Make your way from Steps 2 to 11 without interruption, moving smoothly from area to area. In effect, you are treating the whole body by treating the ear. Energy is directed from the top of the body (head) downward (to the toe) and, thus, is grounded using this technique. This whole process should take approximately 5 minutes. See Figure 6.2 and Figure 6.3 for the directions to massage the ear.

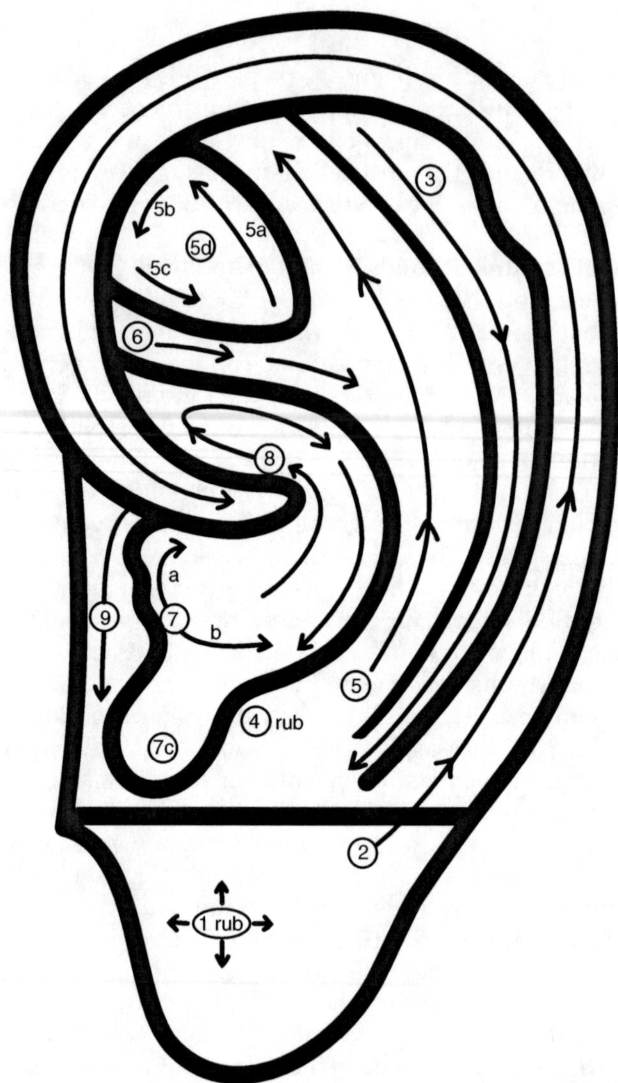

Figure 6.2 Ear massage direction for the anterior aspect of ear.

First, shut off the lights in the room. Sit behind the patient, who is lying supine on the treatment table with eyes closed. Perform all of the ear massage bilaterally and simultaneously.

1. Begin by gently rubbing the patient's ear lobe between your thumb and index finger for about 10 seconds. The thumb rubs the front of the ear and the index finger supports the back of the ear. (*This area corresponds to the head and the face.*)
2. Now make your way up the helix, an area that may feel brittle, crunchy, inflexible. However, it should feel supple. Gently feel each

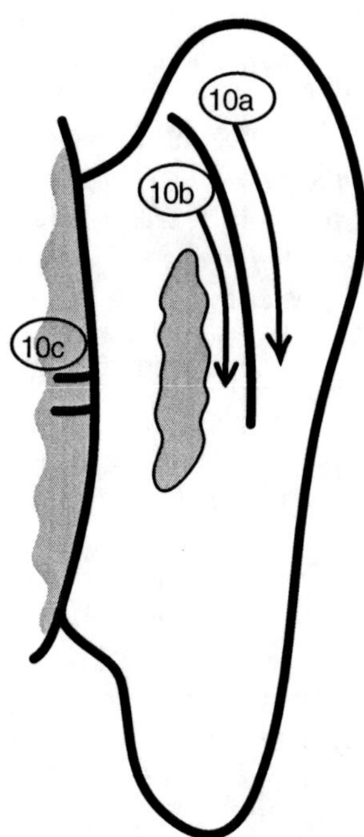

Figure 6.3 Ear massage direction for the posterior aspect of ear.

section of the ear as you proceed from the end of the helix near the lobe all the way around to the crus of the helix. Massage with the thumb and the index finger while simultaneously gently pulling the ear outward. (*This area corresponds to the tonsils and immunity in general.*)

3. Next put your thumb inside the scapha and massage downward toward the lobe. (*This area corresponds to the points of the upper limbs.*)
4. When you get to the lobe, massage the antitragus. Then make your way up the lower antihelix crus and into the superior antihelix crus. (*The antitragus pertains to the brain and nervous regulation; the lower antihelix crus pertains to the structures of the thorax; and the superior antihelix crus to the points of the lower limbs.*)
5. Now go into the triangular fossa, and massage it upward along its superior border, then across and finally downward along its inferior border. Press and hold the center. (*The triangular fossa has a mix of points, many pertaining to hormonal and nervous regulation.*)
6. Put your thumb in the inferior antihelix crus; massage downward, including the spiny portion of the lower antihelix crus. (*The lower antihelix crus relates to additional points in the lower part of the body. The spinal segment pertains to the sacral through cervical vertebrae.*)
7. Now place your thumb in the cavum concha, and rub the points in front of the external auditory meatus. Then follow the border of the supratragic notch. Massage the points in the cavum concha as you

move laterally to the lower antihelix crus. End by pressing at the deepest point of the cavum concha at the level of the intertragic notch. (*These points connect to the organs of the thorax.*)

8. Proceed to the cymba concha and massage sectors 1 to 6 in ascending order. (*These are points pertaining to organs in the lower abdomen.*)
9. Next, massage the points of the tragus in a downward manner. (*These points have a connection to the endocrine system.*)
10. Finally, massage the posterior aspect of the ear. Begin laterally at the hypertension groove and massage downward. Next, massage the areas pertaining to a patient's back in a downward manner and by pressing the vagus point. (*These points regulate blood pressure and treat the back. The vagus point corresponds to the 10th cranial nerve, which regulates many body parts, and digestion and the nervous system, in particular.*)

Apart from generalized ear massage, the vigorous massage of a chosen point can be used to pretest its therapeutic usefulness. For instance, if the patient has a frozen shoulder, vigorously massage the Shoulder point in the ear with a strong dispersive technique by grasping the point firmly between your thumb and index finger and rubbing quickly for about 10 seconds. Simultaneously, instruct the patient to lift and move his or her shoulder. If the practitioner is pressing on the right point and is rubbing it vigorously, the patient, although perhaps wincing, will be able to move the shoulder with almost a full range of motion. This technique is particularly useful for locating precise points to treat musculolskeletal conditions, such as stiff neck, lumbago, arthritic joints, and more. However, this is a powerful technique analogous to needling with a dispersive technique, so prepare the patient for the painful sensation achieved with a strong, dispersive hand technique. Explain that the pain will quickly pass when you stop massaging the point, and this is a better option than surgery, drugs, or other invasive treatments. The simultaneous manipulation of the point by the practitioner, along with the patient lifting and moving the affected area, is critical for therapeutic effectiveness. Many times this is all the treatment that is needed. However, the treatment can be reinforced with needles or continued through take-home therapies, such as pellets and seeds.

Many disorders can be treated through the simple therapy of ear massage. Chen Youbang indicates that "ear massage/press therapy can change anoxia, regulate nonspecific immunity, and strengthen antiinfection effect."[4] This is certainly a simple method that has valuable local and systemic benefits to the human organism.

Needles (2)

In China, needling is the most common ear modality practiced, although seeds are also used. In terms of thickness, the Chinese prefer a thick gauge needle, such as a #28 gauge, in order to obtain a strong *Da Qi* sensation in the ear. Fine needles are likely to bend easily on insertion and may fail to

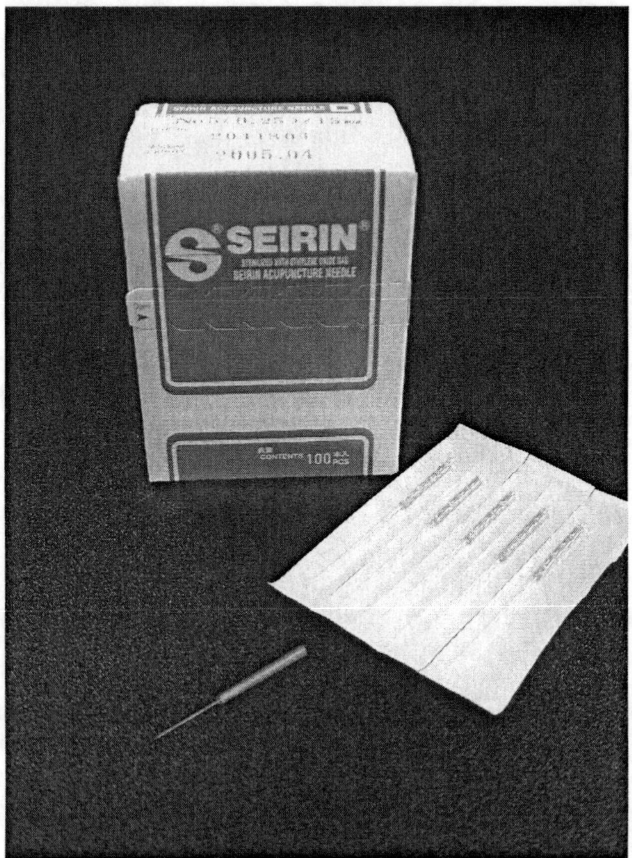

Figure 6.4 Ear needles.

deliver the appropriate needle stimulus. However, if the patient is needle sensitive, if the ear is thin, or if the practitioner has a good needle technique, fine needles, such a #34 or #36 gauge, can work (Figure 6.4).

Short needles, such as half-inch (15 mm), needles should be used since the points in the ear have a shallow depth of insertion. In general, the longer the needle, the more likely it is to fall out because of its weight in relation to the depth of needle insertion. If it falls out, it can tear delicate ear tissue.

To initiate treatment with needles, swipe the patient's ear with an alcohol prep or a cotton ball wet with 70% isopropyl alcohol. You can ask the patient to swipe his or her own ear. This simple step involves the patient in the treatment process, which is a useful treatment strategy. Because of the strength of the ear response when it is treated and the powerful manner in which the *Qi* and Blood are regulated in the ear (with the exception of massage), normally only one ear is needled or treated with any ear modality.

Next, stabilize the patient's ear by supporting the back of the area to be needled with the nondominant hand. Care must be taken not to penetrate through the entire ear with the needle, so feel the thickness of the patient's ear as you prepare to treat. Position the hand holding the needle as closely as possible to the point to be needled. With a half-inch needle, use a free-hand insertion. An insertion tube is not needed for needling ear points all of which have a very shallow depth of about 0.01 in. Freehanded insertion is more accurate in such a small spatial field. When released, the needle should be firmly embedded in the tissue and not left hanging in the ear, which is an improper needling technique that causes pain.

The "secret" to reducing pain either in the ear or in the body begins with the rapid speed of insertion. This swift motion allows for firm penetration of the outermost layer of the skin. The free nerve endings that register pain are embedded in the epidermis or outermost layer of the skin. Slow needling causes pain because the needle lingers through this area. Also, when there is pain, patients typically move to try to get away from it. The skin in the point can then tear as the patient moves from the needle.

After insertion, press the needle slightly into the point and then rotate manually with small amplitude in order to obtain *Qi*. The *Qi* in the ear typically arrives quickly if the ear point location is correct. Various *Da Qi* sensations may be elicited in the ear, but from a clinical standpoint the Chinese maintain that the most desirable sensation in terms of clinical effectiveness is heat. Other sensations, similar to the arrival of *Qi* in the body, include soreness, tingling, referred sensation, numbness, distention, heaviness, awareness of energy, a mild electrical feeling, warmth, mild throbbing, and a spreading or jumping sensation. Patients may be inclined to report that they feel the needling as painful. Indeed, because of the amount of *Qi* converged in the ear as well as the ear's degree of vascularization and innervation, one may be inclined to describe the sensation that way. At this point, you should educate the patient as to the meaning of the feeling; that is, the perception is *Qi* obtained through proper needling vs. pain. Most of the time *Qi* arrival in the ear is strong and swift.

If the *Da Qi* sensation (*Qi* arrival) is not perceived, the angle of insertion of the needle can be adjusted by making it more oblique, directing it upwards or downwards, or medially or laterally. Which direction to alter it is virtually impossible to predict or to standardize. The practitioner is encouraged to practice and develop a proficient needle technique and to gain his or her own experience.

Without delay, as soon as the *Qi* arrives, proceed to tonify or disperse the point depending upon your treatment plan. While David Legge claims that auricular acupuncture tends to have a dispersive technique,[5] others, including myself, would also assert that it is used both to tonify and disperse. Perhaps the best tonification technique in the ear is simply to exert a small twist in a clockwise direction. To disperse, use a more vigorous rotation or turn in a counterclockwise direction. If rotating the needle causes pain (vs. *Qi* arrival), turn the needle the opposite way. In this case, Helmut Kropej recommends rotating the needle once clockwise and once counterclockwise.[6]

If there is persistent pain at the site of needling, remove the needle and consider other points or other methods to use. If a sticking sensation is felt upon needle manipulation, the point is still in need of treatment. Once that tension is relieved or worked out, the affected part is considered treated. Often during treatment the needle that was originally firmly in place falls out of the point. What has occurred is that the *Qi* has expelled the needle from the ear. This means that the work of the needle has been accomplished.

Due to its rich vascularization, the ear may bleed easily when needled. If bleeding occurs, allow the ear to bleed instead of trying to stop the flow. Absorb the droplets with a sterile cotton ball. Wear gloves to guard against the transmission of blood-borne pathogens. Purposeful ear bleeding is an ear acupuncture technique that is discussed later in this chapter.

A small number of needles are often sufficient to produce decisive results in treatment. Several needles are sometimes inserted into the same point for added therapeutic effect. Some practitioners let their patients leave the office with an ear needle in place. In that case they need to be told what to do in the event of ear bleeding and how to dispose of the needle properly. This is not a technique that I employ or advocate, as there are numerous other take-home modalities from which to choose.

Needles are typically retained for 15 to 20 minutes. However, in acute cases, needles may be left in for several hours without depleting the body's energy. As a clinical tip, due to its soft composition, I prefer not to needle the ear lobe. The needle is not as well retained in the lobe as it is in the cartilage or in the connective tissue of the upper aspect of the ear, so other modalities can be selected to treat points on the ear lobe.

Ear seeds and herbal plasters (3)

In contemporary China, ear seeds are a standard way in which most auriculotherapy is administered for virtually every treatable condition. The most commonly used seeds, semen vaccaria or cow's herd seeds, are not chosen for external use due to any inherent medicinal property. Rather, these seeds are chosen because they are plentiful, inexpensive, and of appropriate size and density to deliver a strong stimulus when pressed (Figure 6.5). Recently, sterilized semen vaccaria seeds attached to adhesives (called ear plasters) have become commercially available for ease of administration. If you use loose (bulk) ear seeds, take care to sterilize the seeds before use; otherwise infection can ensue from dirty, unsterile seeds. Then place tape over the seed to secure it in the ear. Sometimes in China mustard, radish, or perilla seeds are used.

Ear seeds can be attached to all points in the ear. An effective technique to reinforce a point is to place one seed on the anterior surface of the ear and put another exactly opposite it on the posterior surface. In this way, when they are rubbed, a stronger stimulus is delivered through the heat produced by friction.

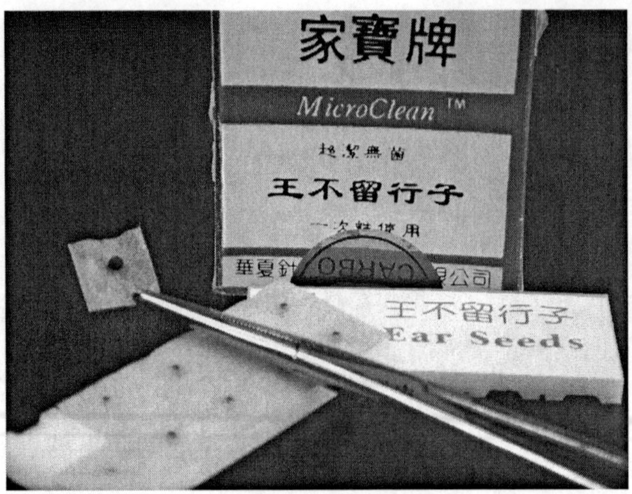

Figure 6.5 Ear seeds.

To apply the ear plaster, pick up the plaster with a pair forceps or tweezers and affix it to the ear that has been previously cleaned with alcohol and allowed to dry. The average retention time of the seeds is 3 to 5 days, as long as they do not become wet or humidity levels become too high. Instruct the patient to keep the ear seeds dry by covering the ear with a towel or shower cap when washing or showering. Seeds should be removed if the stimulus becomes too painful or if the ear feels irritated. Patients are instructed to press on the seeds 3 to 5 times a day for 3 to 5 seconds at a time. To remove the seeds, the patient just needs to peel back the tape and the seed should follow.

On occasion, seeds are dipped in particular medicinal substances, such as placenta or other herbs, and applied to the ear in the same manner. This method has the added therapeutic benefit of conferring the healing effects of the herbs as well as the benefits of ear treatment.[7] Additional substances include mashed garlic and black pepper, fresh mashed ginger and pepper, and others.[8]

Clinical notes

- **Note 1** — "The authors corrected the abnormal fetal position in 413 cases of pregnant women by the auricular-plaster therapy with a success rate of 83.3%; remarkably higher than treatment by knee-chest positioning."[9]
- **Note 2** — "To relieve the discomfort due to gastrointestinal dysfunction following abdominal operations, auricular-plaster therapy (in combination with ST 36 [*Zusanli*]) restored normal peristalsis within 72 hours in over 92% of the cases involved. This was compared with a 46% rate in a control group suggesting that this combined method may promote postoperative recovery of intestinal function."[10]

Ear pellets (4)

Ear pellets (or BBs) are a convenient method for administering an ear acupuncture treatment (Figure 6.6). It is my favorite method of ear delivery. The BBs come in sterile silver, gold, titanium, copper, and stainless steel. They are affixed to either clear or flesh colored plasters that can easily be applied to the ear by picking up the BB with tweezers or forceps. The size of the BB is perfect for discrete stimulation of the point and almost unnoticeable in the ear.

Points that are indicative of a deficiency require gold for treatment, whereas those indicating an excess necessitate silver. Use gold for pain from exhaustion, hypofunction, or pain that increases when the specific action of the auricular point is called into function. Silver is used for pain caused by hyperfunction, trauma, or pain that increases at rest and improves with movement. If you are not sure what metal to choose, palpate the points with an ear probe. If the pain created by contact with the probe radiates over a large area of the ear, an excess condition of hyperfunction is indicated and silver will disperse the pain. If the pain only radiates over a limited area, use gold. I have no clinical experience with stainless steel, copper, or titanium BBs. Stainless steel and titanium pellets have a neutral, balancing property and can be used either way with the therapeutic action achieved via the stimulus vs. the quality of the metal.

Helmut Kropej notes in discussing the metallurgic properties of needles that "although there is no definitive scientific proof as yet to the different effects of gold and silver needles, we can state that the action of precious metals is based on their own electrical potential. Gold has an electrical potential of +0.285 and silver of only –0.048 on the basis of the hydrogen electrode. This potential is, however, increased by the contact potential after insertion of the needle into the tissue, resulting in an even greater potential difference."[11]

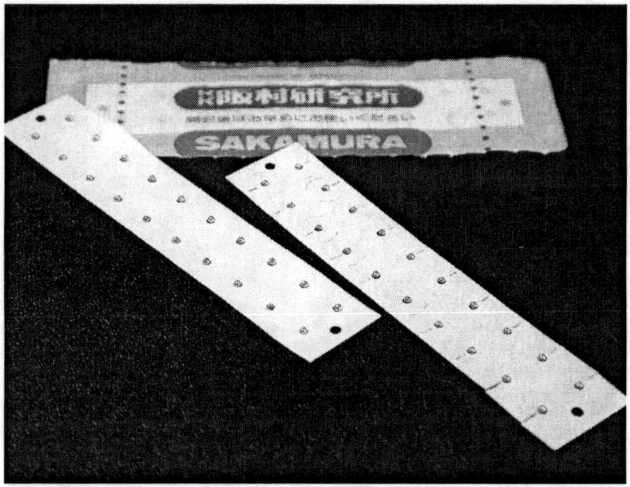

Figure 6.6 Ear pellets.

He also says that, "in contrast to body acupuncture, incorrect selection of the metal of the needle manifests itself in the ear with immediate intensification of the peripheral complaints. This is the result of ear acupuncture reflex action. The error can be corrected by using a different metal."[11] The same can be said of ear pellets.

The practioner should provide the same instructions to patients in regard to retention time for the pellets, how to press, how frequently, how long, and also to keep the area dry.

Ear tacks (5)

Ear tacks are another modality that is somewhat similar to seeds and pellets. They look like small thumb tacks and come in several sizes: extra small, small, medium, and large. In general, the bigger the tack the stronger the stimulus obtained in the ear. Extra small or small-size tacks seem to be the most comfortable for patients, yet still offer a suitable stimulus. The tacks come affixed to flesh colored tape and can be applied to the ear with tweezers or forceps (Figure 6.7).

Because ear tacks pierce the skin, only retain them in the ear for a limited amount of time so that infection does not occur. The typical retention time is theoretically 3 to 5 days. Because their stimulus is so strong, a few hours to a day may be all that the patient can tolerate. Exposure to water through swimming, bathing, or high humidity levels can increase the risk of infection. Inquire about the patient's lifestyle (for instance, does he swim frequently, etc.), and adjust the tack retention time accordingly. The ear normally replaces its epithelium about every 5 days, so sometimes the needle may be automatically extruded.

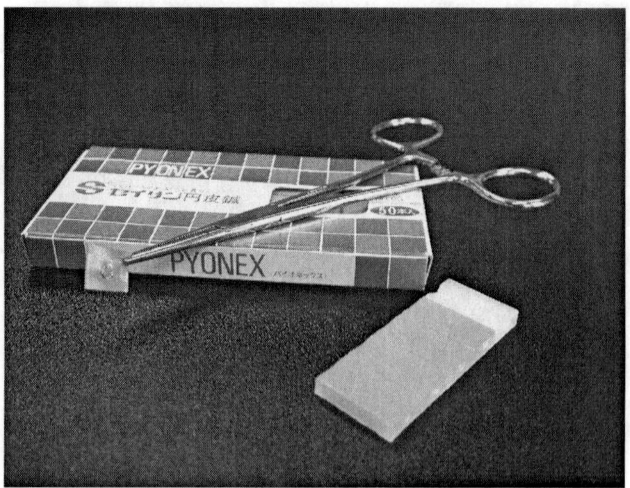

Figure 6.7 Ear tacks.

Table 6.2 Home Care for Your Ear Treatment

Ear acupressure treatments include the placement of pellets, seeds, or tacks on specific points of the ear to prevent or to treat disease or pain. They may be used as an adjunct to regular acupuncture treatments, used to enhance and prolong its effects, or used alone as the primary form of treatment. Ear treatment is an important aspect of healthcare. In order to ensure optimal results, please follow the guidelines detailed below:

1. Press gently and rhythmically on the ear pellet, seed, or tack 3 to 5 times a day for several seconds. This should produce a mild sensation of heat, distention, heaviness, or soreness. The sensation is a sign that the treatment is working. Do not press for longer than 3 to 5 seconds each time as irritation may develop.
2. When bathing or swimming, it is important not to get the ear wet. Wrap a towel around your head or use a shower cap that tightly covers the ear. A cotton ball loosely placed in the ear is also helpful when you shower.
3. All ear therapies should be replaced every 3 to 5 days. This not only ensures the best results, but also protects the ear against infection. It is important that you follow your practitioner's advice on when to return to the office to have the ear therapy changed.
4. Important note: If the ear therapy becomes too painful, carefully peel back the tape. The tape will come off along with the seed, pellet, or tac. If the ear therapy comes off accidentally, do not attempt to replace it yourself (unless you are sure where it goes), as you may place it on an incorrect point.
5. When removing the ear therapy, some bleeding may occur, although this should not happen unless you have been pressing too hard on the point. Be prepared for this by having a cotton ball in your hand as you remove the tac, seed, or pellet. Press the point lightly to absorb the blood, and then dispose of the blood-tinged cotton ball in the garbage. If someone else is removing your therapy, they should wear disposable gloves to guard against infection that can be transmitted through the blood.
6. The diagram (Figure 6.8) shows the location of your ear therapy. You have _____ seeds, tacks, pellets in your ear.

If you have any questions, please do not hesitate to contact your practitioner.

Patients should be given a similar instruction sheet (Table 6.2) to educate them about ear therapy, to encourage their compliance with the modality, and ensure their safety.

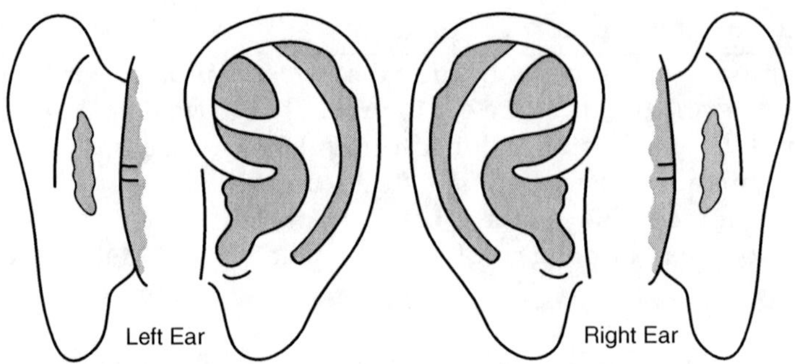

Figure 6.8 Ear therapy illustrated in the left and right ear.

Intradermal needles (6)

Intradermals are small fine needles that can be embedded in a point or an area (Figure 6.9). They are an excellent choice for threading (i.e., connecting) points in the ear. The most common areas for intradermal needle use are points that are large or on an area such as the Constipation area or various vertebral segments.

Intradermal needles are sterile and come in various lengths. The most common lengths are 3 and 6 mm, with the longer needle indicated by the higher number. Choose the size which best fits the affected area.

Before inserting the intradermal needle, clean the ear with alcohol and allow the ear to dry naturally. Peel back the packaging of the needle and pick up the needle with your tweezers or forceps positioned at a 90° angle to the needle. This angle allows you to easily insert the needle into the point. The needle can then be covered with a small piece of tape to keep it from

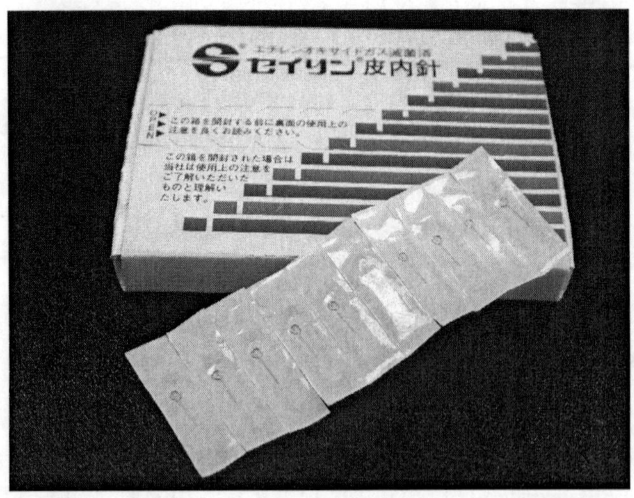

Figure 6.9 Intradermal needles.

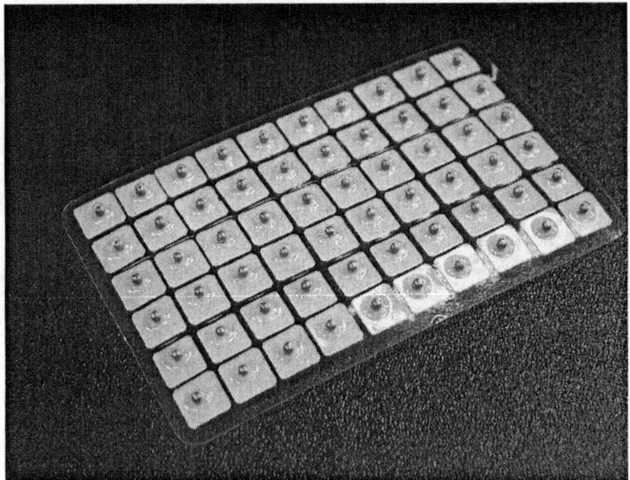

Figure 6.10 Ear magnets.

bending, falling out, or getting wet, which could lead to infection. Intradermals may be "piggybacked" (i.e., arranged back to back) in order to treat an area such as the lumbar vertebrae.

If comfortable, leave the needle in for 2 to 5 days, then have the patient return to you for removal. Because intradermals are implanted subcutaneously, they must be pulled out in a particular direction Thus, the main disadvantage of an interdermal needle is that its use necessitates that the patient return to the office within 3 to 5 days, or earlier if the patient experiences any discomfort.

Magnets (7)

Magnets are a modern and effective method of auricular treatment administration (Figure 6.10). They are comfortable to wear, do not pierce the skin, and can be removed at bedtime or as needed due to symptoms such as discomfort. There are different sizes and types of ear magnets, so consult the manufacturer's instructions for product use. Magnet therapy instructions should be provided to patients (Table 6.3). There are some contraindications to magnet use and these are described in the Home Care for Magnet Therapy form.

Electricity (8)

Electricity is one of the most common methods used in auricular medicine. Many research studies relate to the use of electroacupuncture for the detection and treatment of illness. Many healthcare professionals use electric stimulation for both diagnosis and treatment of the patient. However, I personally do not like using electrical machines for treatment. There are

Table 6.3 Home Care for Magnet Therapy

- Your practitioner has prescribed ___ magnets for you. Wear these for 4 to 6 hours during the day for as long as prescribed by the practioner. Remove the magnets if they are in any way uncomfortable. If you have a pacemaker, defibrillator, ear implants, are pregnant, or have any metal implants in your body, you should *not* use magnets. Do *not* wear magnets if you are sensitive to electromagnetism or are an epileptic. Remove all jewelry when wearing magnets, especially ear jewelry. If your symptoms worsen, remove the magnets. Never wear the magnets to bed, as they may fall off, stick to a different or inappropriate ear point, or fall into the ear canal. Remove magnets before receiving x-rays, MRIs, or other similar diagnostic techniques. Magnets are for single patient use. Do not share or trade magnets with other people.

If you have any questions or problems, please contact your practitioner.

voluminous journal articles and books, which expertly discuss this modality in depth. A considerable number of these can be found in the bibliographies listed at the end of each chapter.

If you have an electrical acupuncture machine with a point detector, such as an AWQ 100B, you may use the probe to scan the ear. Do *not* swab the ear with alcohol prior to performing this step, as the alcohol removes pathology in the ear, such as suppurations, and changes the electrical potential in the ear, which is what the electrical apparatus is trying to detect.

Scanning of the ear can be used diagnostically for detection of possible pathology. Low electrical resistance, or inversely stated, increased (higher) conductivity can be detected on acupuncture points on the body and on the ear. When pathology develops, the auricular point representing the diseased organ or body part has an even higher degree of electrodermal activity. This increase in conductivity registers with the electrical machine as a beep. Katsusuke Serizawa explains, "Studies on the response of the viscera to auricular points have shown that a change in electroconductivity of corresponding auricular points may be induced by a pathological change in certain regions of the organism. The extent of this response is directly proportional to the degree of the seriousness of the disease."[12] Interestingly, Joseph Helms writes that "electrical instrumentation does not distinguish between old and new problems. However, pain is most likely to be an added characteristic for the active point."[13]

As you systematically touch the points in the ear, carefully apply equal pressure or the points may register differently. If an area is pressed repeatedly, changes in electrical resistance develop. Other factors, such as age, weather, excess perspiration, excess wax accumulation, and even a history of working indoors, affects the electrical resistance in the ear. For these reasons, electricity is not my preferred method of treatment.

Electroacupuncture is absolutely contraindicated for patients with pacemakers, as electroacupuncture has been shown to electromagnetically interfere with the pacemaker function. Electroacupuncture should not be used on patients who cannot tolerate a strong stimulus. To achieve an anesthetizing effect, electroacupuncture is the modality of choice. How to use electroacupuncture for anesthetization is beyond the scope of this discussion.

Bleeding (9)

Bleeding is an effective ear modality when applied to certain ear points. The therapeutic effects of bleeding are fourfold:

1. Reduces excess Heat and Fire
2. Brings down *Yang*
3. Stimulates *Qi* and Blood flow
4. Moves Stagnant *Qi* and Blood

Ear points may be bled when these strategies are required. Specifically, the Hypertension points in the ear may be bled if the patient's type of high blood pressure is an excess type, such as Liver *Yang* Rising with Heat. High blood pressure due to Kidney *Yin* Deficiency would not benefit from this type of modality and, in fact, could weaken the patient. Ear points, which exhibit signs of Blood Stagnation, such as petechiae or red spots, may be bled. For instance, a red spot on the Upper Lung point may appear when the patient has a sore throat. It could be bled to relieve the sore throat. Certain points, such as *Shenmen* and Occiput, are more likely to bleed than others. This method is contraindicated for patients with a history of bleeding disorders. Keep in mind that the ears of patients with high blood pressure may bleed more easily than those with normal blood pressure.

Position the patient in a reclining position to bleed. Gloves are worn by the practitioner for protection from contact with the patient's blood. Massage the ear to promote capillary congestion, which will assist in bleeding by increasing blood flow to the ear. Select a regular 28-gauge, half-inch acupuncture needle, just like the needle used for ear acupuncture. Medical lancets, which are sometimes used to bleed body acupuncture points, are too big, will induce too much bleeding, and increase the chance of infection of the ear. Puncture quickly and to the same depth as the recommended needling (0.01 in.). Absorb the droplets of blood elicited by placing a cotton ball over the point and pressing lightly. This small amount of blood-tinged cotton may be disposed of in the garbage basket. Do *not* bleed more than three points at a time; bleeding one point is the norm and is often sufficient.

Clinical notes

Note 3 — "Chinese clinical studies, particularly in the areas of treating infantile tetany, infantile epilepsy, and headache have shown that bleeding therapy is an effective modality. It can be applied to the capillaries on the dorsum of the ear to reduce the pathogenic evil from all the *Yang* meridians, and promote the function of resuscitation, sedation, analgesia, and relaxation."[14]

Moxibustion (10)

Moxa provides the powerful therapeutic effects of tonifying the *Qi* and *Yang*, removing Cold, and increasing the flow of *Qi* and Blood in the channels. Generally speaking, moxa is not used for most points in the ear due to the relatively small size of the ear points and the large size of most moxa instruments. Incense stick-size moxa is convenient in treating such small points. Hold a moxa stick over the Common Cold point to treat a cold or, preventatively, to deter a cold. If needles are inserted in the ear, a moxa stick may be held over the needle handle to conduct heat into the point. Facial paralysis, ophthalmic pain, mumps, painful *bi* syndromes painful obstruction, herpes zoster, and auricular chondritis are well treated with auricular moxibustion. Moxa smoke can be blown into the ear to treat earache.

Incisions and sutures (11)

Incisions are an old Chinese technique whereby small cuts are made into the skin of the ear in order to "activate" the function of the point. This method is sometimes called auricular scratching or cutting therapy. The healing mechanism initiated by the incision is the same mechanism that stimulates the incised point. Sometimes herbal substances are implanted into the cut to confer the therapeutic properties of the herbs. This treatment method falls into the area of surgery. It is too drastic for most patients and conditions and is not legal for most acupuncturists to perform. (Consult the scope of practice that applies to your state.)

Low used a similar technique involving sutures for the management of withdrawal symptoms. With this technique, catgut, along with nylon thread and a steel bead, was implanted to stimulate the point. This method is somewhat radical and, likewise, would be construed as surgery. Chances of infection are increased with these invasive methods.

Injections (12)

Injections are a possible method of ear therapy. Injections involve the administration of various substances into acupuncture points to stimulate the physiological functions of the points through the pharmacological properties of the injected substances. Common injectables include saline (which simply stimulates the point); vitamin B_{12} (for nerve enrichment); lidocaine and procaine (for pain); placenta (to nourish *Qi*, Blood, and Essence); various Chinese herbal solutions, such as carthamus and ligustrum (most of which have the property of moving *Qi* and Blood); and homeopathic substances for their specific properties. A disadvantage of ear injections is the pain caused from the size of the hypodermic needle in relation to the size of the ear, as well as the pain caused by the injected substance (particularly alcohol), which is in the Chinese injections.

Clinical notes

Note 4 — "In treating functional bleeding of the uterus, small amounts of vitamin K_3 were injected into the Diaphragm point. The Diaphragm point was chosen because in traditional theory, the diaphragm is the point where the Blood meets and can be directed to the proper meridians. Therefore, that point is indicated for treating diseases caused by bleeding due to Evil Heat in the Blood. Vitamin K_3 promotes circulation and removal of Blood Stasis and lets the Blood go back to its original meridian. The Uterus point was injected with 0.1 ml of vitamin K_3 with a 1 ml syringe and #5 g needle. The procedure was repeated every 3 to 4 days. The total success rate was 97% with results ranging from full recovery (48 cases), marked recovery (12 cases), some alleviation (8 cases), and unsuccessful (2 cases). The majority of patients experienced a general decrease in bleeding after the initial treatment, a marked decrease after the second treatment, and bleeding was eventually checked after the third or fourth treatment. Follow-up observation found no reoccurrence in most cases and a return to normal menses.[15]

Laser (13)

The cold laser has been found useful for conditions treatable through the ear. Since the laser is a form of light therapy, the laser does not pierce the skin, infection and cellulitis issues are essentially moot, and the therapy is painless. In addition, the laser can precisely target the point. Because of these features, more investigation into the use of laser auriculotherapy merits consideration.

Clinical notes

Note 5 — "A 1990 study showed that treatment with the helium-neon auriculotherapy laser can increase the experimental pain threshold and suggests a possible alternative for patients intolerant of transcutaneous electrical nerve stimulation."[16]

Staples (14)

Staplepuncture is a technique that was used in early studies on auriculotherapy. Sacks developed the staple acupuncture technique. With this modality, a surgical staple is placed in the ear, thus allowing for the puncture of two points. Sacks maintained that the staples could safely be retained in the ear for 2 weeks. This procedure is analogous to incisions and sutures in terms of its invasiveness and would be considered a surgical procedure today.

Plum blossom needling (15)

Plum blossom needling therapy of the auricle is sometimes used to induce bleeding for the various therapeutic usages of bleeding. Care must be taken to protect the auricle from infection with this method when one selects the plum blossum needle, a hammerlike tool, to tap the ear, as infection could develop when the small holes are produced in the ear skin. Points on the lobe are most commonly treated with this method.

Which side of the ear to treat?

There are no hard and fast rules regarding which side of the ear on which to begin treatment. Ultimately, the goal is to simply treat in the most effective manner possible. However, since one needs a starting place, the following guidelines are offered:

1. If a problem is not confined to one particular side (for instance, the patient has insomnia or a menstrual disorder vs. a right-sided shoulder problem), treat the right ear in a woman and the left ear in a man. This treatment protocol corresponds to gender in Oriental medicine where the right side and females are considered *Yin* and the left side and males are *Yang*. Use this approach provided there is no surface or visible pathology that would contraindicate treatment; for instance, a rash or skin irritation on that side of the ear that would preclude treatment at that location.
2. If the problem is musculoskeletal or pertains to a particular side of the body, treat the same ear as the side the problem is manifested on. For instance, if a patient has right-sided knee pain, treat the right ear. However, there are times when the opposite ear works better. For instance, a patient may have left shoulder pain in the area of LI 15 (*Jianyu*). Because the Large Intestine meridian's divergent channel exits from LI 15 and crosses as it traverses to the face, the right ear may be more effective. This style of needling, called contralateral needling, is useful in both body and ear acupuncture.
3. After treating the patient with needles in one ear during a session, you then choose to affix pellets or other modalities to reinforce that treatment for take-home purposes, treat the opposite ear so as not to irritate the ear that was needled.
4. Consider patient lifestyle variables or the condition of the ear, for example, if the patient sleeps exclusively on one side of the body, has a job talking on the phone for long periods and primarily uses one ear, or has a hearing aid, multiple earpiercing, or jewelry that is

difficult to remove. Select the opposite ear to treat in these cases or do not treat at all.
5. When the patient returns for the next treatment in a series, alternate ears and use the opposite ear in order to reduce irritation and chances of infection.

Therapeutic result

With all of the auriculotherapy modalities outlined, the following therapeutic outcomes can occur:

1. The complaint and its manifestations or pain may disappear in seconds.
2. The problem may take a few days to resolve if the disorder is an organ problem.
3. The condition may worsen in sensitive patients. Depending upon the symptoms, this aggravation may constitute a healing crisis or the therapy may not be suitable for the patient.
4. Acute disorders tend to improve faster than chronic ones.
5. Endocrine disorders are most likely interrelated; hence, several points that affect the endocrine system are required in a prescription.
6. Diseases of the *Yang* organs tend to heal faster than the *Yin* organs. Because *Yin* organs are solid in nature, they are more difficult to heal.
7. Regardless of the modality chosen, the patient can feel tired after treatment. Allow the patient to rest in your office so he does not leave in a mentally or physically drained condition.

Auriculotherapy is one of my favorite methods for treating the elderly or those who like added reinforcement and/or extended benefit from treatment, as well as for the treatment of musculoskeletal and internal organ problems.

"According to a series of analyses of therapeutic results of 14,886 cases, ear needling was found to be effective in 90.1% of cases," writes Katsusuke Serizawa.[17] As has been discussed, if there is a corresponding body part that is impaired, such as the knee or shoulder, and that part is mobilized simultaneously with the vigorous massage or needling of the point, the therapeutic effect is even better.

References

1. Nogier, P. *Handbook of Auriculotherapy.* Maisonneuve, Moulins-les–Metz, France, 1981, p. 119.
2. Huang, H. *Auriculotherapy Diagnosis and Treatment*. Longevity Press, Bellaire, TX, 1996, p. 286.
3. Bartnett, B. *Auricular Therapy – Theory and Practice.* Ruidoso Health Institute, Ruidoso, NM, 1999, p. 66.
4. Youbang, C. and Liangyue, D., Eds. *Essentials of Contemporary Chinese Acupuncturists' Clinical Experiences.* Foreign Language Press, Beijing, 1989, p. 217.

5. Legge, D. *Close to the Bone: The Treatment of Musculoskeletal Disorder with Acupuncture and other Traditional Chinese Medicine*. Sydney College Press, Australia, 1990, p. 292.
6. Kropej, H. *The Fundamentals of Ear Acupuncture, 4th ed.* Karl F. Haug Publishers, Heidelberg, Germany; 1991, p. 22.
7. Liu, H., Lu, Y., Dong, Q., and Zhong, X. Treatment of adolescent myopia by pressure plaster of semen impatientis on otopoiunts. *J. Trad. Chin. Med.*, Dec. 1991, 14(4): 283–286; and Yang, C. et al. 268 cases of myopia treated with injection and pellet pressure at auriculopoints. *J. Trad. Chin. Med.*, Sept. 1993, 13(3): 196.
8. Huang, H. *Auriculotherapy Diagnosis and Treatment*. Longevity Press, Bellaire, TX, 1996, p. 271.
9. Qin, G.F. 413 cases of abnormal fetal position corrected by auricular plaster therapy. *J. Trad. Chin. Med.*, Dec. 1989, 9(4): 235–237.
10. Wan, Q. Auricular-plaster therapy plus acupuncture at zusanli for postoperative recovery of intestinal function. *J. Trad. Chin. Med.*, 2000 Jun., 20(2): 134–136.
11. Kropej, H. *The Fundamentals of Ear Acupuncture, 4th ed.* Karl F. Haug Publishers, Heidelberg, Germany; 1991, p. 22.
12. Serizawa, K. *Clinical Acupuncture, A Practical Japanese Approach.* Japan Publications, Tokyo, 1988, pp. 112, 114.
13. Helms, J. *Acupuncture Energetics: A Clinical Approach for Physicians.* Medical Acupuncture Publishers, Berkeley, CA, 1995, p. 140.
14. Serizawa, K. *Clinical Acupuncture, A Practical Japanese Approach.* Japan Publications, Tokyo, 1988, p. 237.
15. Niu, M. *Functional Bleeding of Uterus with Auriculoacupuncture*. Department of TCM, Dezhou District Hospital, Shendong, China, 2001.
16. King, C.E., Clelland, J.A., Knowles, C.J. et al. Effect of helium-neon laser auriculotherapy on experimental pain threshold. *Phys. Ther.*, 1990, 70(1): 24–30.
17. Serizawa, K. *Clinical Acupuncture, A Practical Japanese Approach.* Japan Publications, Tokyo, 1988, p. 444.

Bibliography

Alimi, D., Rubino, C., Leandri, E.P., and Brule, S.F. Analgesic effects of auricular acupuncture for cancer pain. *J. Pain Symptom. Manage.*, 2000 Feb. 19(2): 81–82.

Bartnett, B. Ear massage. *Massage*, #345, Sept./Oct. 1993.

Bartnett, B. *Auricular Therapy – Theory and Practice.* Ruidoso Health Institute, Ruidoso, NM, 1999.

Bragin, E.O., Dionne, R. Moody, T., and Pert, K. Changes in the content of opiate-like substances in auricular electroacupuncture anesthesia of rats. *Vopr. Med. Khim.*, Jul.–Aug. 1982, 28(4): 102–105, (in Russian).

Bragin, E.O., Vasilenko, G.F., Batueva, N.N., Belitskaia, R.A., and Shumova, O.V. The role of catecholaminergi group–A5 neurons in analgesia induced by auricular electroacupuncture and in electrodermal pain stimulation. *Biull. Eksp. Bio. Med.*, Mar. 1989, 107(3): 310–312, (in Russian).

Brule–Fermand, S. Treatment of chronic cancer pain. Contribution of acupuncture, auriculotherapy, and mesotherapy. *Soins*, Jan. 1993, 5568: 39–40, (in French).

Caracausi, S.R. and Lorenzini, R. Ear acupuncture – a modified method – in surgery for 'high risk' patients. *Acta Anasthesiol.*, 1977, 28(5): 721–730, (in Italian).

Caracausi, S.R., Lorenzini, R., Pilloni, C., Tognali, F., and Sciaretta, G. Spectrum analysis of the electroencephalogram during electrohypoalgesia (combined with electroacupuncture) and pharmacological anesthesia. *Minerva Med.*, Sept. 15, 1981, 72(33): 2209–2214 (in Italian).

Ceccherelli, F., Gagliardi, G., Seda, R., Corradin, M., and Giron, G. Different analgesic effects of manual and electrical acupuncture stimulation of real and sham auricular points: a blind controlled study with rats. *Acupunc. Electrother. Res.*, 1999, 24(3–4): 169–179.

Chen, H. and Ma, Y. Treatment of juvenile ametropia by auricular-plaster therapy combined with plum-blossom needle tapping – a report of 200 cases. *J. Trad. Chin. Med.*, 1998 Mar., 18(1): 47–48.

Chen, J.H. and Guo, J.S. Acupuncture-moxibustion treatment of 30 cases of simple obesity. *Clin. J. Chin. Med.*, 1984, 5(4): 79.

Chen, K., Zhou, S., and Zhao, Y. Auriculoacupuncture therapy – a traditional Chinese method of treatment. *J. Trad. Chin. Med.*, Sept. 1992, 12(3): 233–235.

Chen, K., Zhou, S., and Zheng, Y. Clinical application of traditional auriculoacupoint therapy. *J. Trad. Chin. Med.*, Jun., 1993, 13(2): 152–154.

Cheng, H.F. Ear point pressure with herbal medicine for treating myopia in youngsters. *Chin. Acupunc. Moxibustion*, Feb. 1988, 8(1): 22.

Cheng, H. Treatment of juvenile ametropia by auricular-plaster therapy combined w/plum-blossom needle tapping. *J. Trad. Chin. Med.*, Mar. 1998, 18(1): 47–48.

Choy, D.S. Effect of tragus clips on gastric peristalsis: a pilot study. *J. Altern. Compl. Ther.*, Winter 1998, 4(4): 399–403.

Chun, S. and Heather, A.J. Auriculotherapy: micro-current application on the ear. Clinical pilot study on 57 chronic pain syndromes. *Am. J. Chin. Med.*, 1974, 2(4): 399–405.

Debreceni, L. The effect of electrical stimulation of the ear points on the plasma ACTH and GH level in human. *Acupunc. Electrother. Res.*, 1991, 16(1–2): 45–51.

Dillon, M. and Lucas, C. Auricular stud acupuncture in palliative care patients. *Palliat. Med.*, May 1999, 13(3): 253–254.

Donose, B. et al. *Auricular Inferential Electroanalgesia in Stomatology.* Paper presented at the International Medical Acupuncture Conference, London, May 4–8, 1986.

Fedoseeva, O.V., Kalyuzhnyi, L.V., and Sudakov, K.V. New peptide mechanism of auriculo-acupuncture electro-analgesia: role of angiotensin II. *Acupunc. Electrother. Res.*, 1990, 15(1): 1–8.

Fung, K.P., Choa, G.H., Choy, Y.M., Lee, C.Y., Leung, K.C., Tsang, D., Tso, W.W., and Wen, H.L. Effect of electro-acupuncture on behavioral responses and plasma levels of ACTH and TSH in naloxone-induced morphine withdrawal in rats. *Am. J. Chin. Med.*, Spring–Summer 1980, 8(1–2): 167–169.

Garkavenko, V.V., Vaschenko, E.A., and Limanskii, I.P. Changes in somatosensory evoked potentials in patients with vertebrogenic pain syndromes treated by electroacupuncture. *Fiziol. ZH*, 1989 May–Jun., 35(3): 12–16, (in Russian).

Guan, Z.X. General introduction to the ear point staining method. *Chin. Acupunc. Moxibustion*, Aug. 1986, 6(4): 31–33.

Guo, W. and Zhu, H. Clinical observation in treating 32 diabetic patients with ear-point plaster therapy. *Int. J. Clin. Acupunc.*, 1993, 4(1): 97–99.

Han, J.S., Li, S.J., and Tang, J. Tolerance to electroacupuncture and its cross tolerance to morphine. *Neuropharmacology*, Jun. 1981, 20(6): 593–596.

Han, J.S. and Zhang, R.L. Suppression of morphine abstinence syndrome by body electroacupuncture of different frequencies in rats. *Drug Alc. Depend.*, 1993, 31(2): 169–176.

Huang, H. *Auriculotherapy Diagnosis and Treatment* Longevity Press, Bellaire, TX, 1996.

Hsu, E. Innovations in acumoxa: acupuncture analgesia, scalp and ear acupuncture in the People's Republic of China. *Soc. Sci. Med.*, Feb. 1966, 42(3): 421–430.

Ishchenko, A.N., Zubkov, P.I., Kornev, V.A., and Shev'ev, P.P. A device based on the single-crystal microcomputers for auricular diagnosis and therapy. *Med. Tekh.*, Mar.–Apr. 1990, 2: 25–27, (in Russian).

Jiang, J. Clinical study and application of auricular magnet anesthesia for the operation of the thyroid. *Zhen Ci Yan Jiu*, 1995, 20(3): 4–8, (in Chinese).

King, C.E., Clelland, J.A., Knowles, C.J. et al. Effect of helium-neon laser auriculotherapy on experimental pain threshold. *Phys. Ther.*, 1990, 70(1): 24–30.

Kropej, H. *The Fundamentals of Ear Acupuncture, 4th ed.* Karl F. Haug Publishers, Heidelberg, Germany, 1991.

Lee, T.N. Lidocaine injection of auricular points in treatment of insomnia. *Am. J. Chin. Med.*, Spring 1977, 5(1): 71–77.

Legge, D. *Close to the Bone: The Treatment of Musculoskeletal Disorder with Acupuncture and other Traditional Chinese Medicine.* Sydney College Press, Australia, 1990.

Liu, H., Lu, Y., Dong, Q., and Zhong, X. Treatment of adolescent myopia by pressure plaster of semen impatientis on otopoints. *J. Trad. Chin. Med.*, Dec. 1991, 14(4): 283–286; and Yang, C. et al. 268 cases of myopia treated with injection and pellet pressure at auriculopoints. *J. Trad. Chin. Med.*, Sept. 1993, 13(3).

Low, S.A. Acupuncture and heroin withdrawal. *Med. J. Aust.*, 1974, 31, 3(9): 341.

Luo, H.C. et al. Electroacupuncture vs. amitriptyline in the treatment of depressive states. *J. Trad. Chin. Med.*, 1985, 5: 3.

Masala, A., Satta, G., Alagna, S., Zolo, T.A., Rovasion, P.P., and Rassu, S. Suppression of electroacupuncture (EA)–induced beta-endorphin and ACTH release by hydrocortisone in man. Absence of effects on EA–induced anesthesia. *Acta Endocrinol.*, Aug. 1983, 103(4): 469–472, (in Danish).

Mustafin, A.M. The connection between the biologically active points of the skin and physiological functions. *Biull. Eksp. Biol. Med.*, Jul. 1993, 116(7s): 100–101, (in Russian).

Nikolaev, N.A. Therapeutic effectiveness of laser and EAP in early cerebral-circulation insufficiency. *Am. J. Acupunc.*, 1986, (Abs.) 14: 179; ex. *Zh. Nevropatol. Psikhiatrii*, 1986; 86: 60–64 (in Russian).

Nogier, P. *Handbook of Auriculotherapy.* Maisonneuve, Moulins-les–Metz, France, 1981.

Park, J., White, A., and Ernst, E. New sham method in auricular medicine. *Arch. Intern. Med.*, Mar. 26, 2001, 161(6): 894.

Qin, G.F. 413 cases of abnormal fetal position corrected by auricular plaster therapy. *J. Trad. Chin. Med.*, Dec. 1989, 9(4).

Serizawa, K. *Clinical Acupuncture, A Practical Japanese Approach.* Japan Publications, Tokyo, 1988, pp. 112, 114.

Shapiro, R.S. Rapid effective, non-invasive treatment of pain and disease with acupuncture magnets. *Am. J. Acupunc.*, 1987, 15(1): 43–47.

Shapiro, R.S., Christopher, W., and Cicora, B. Effective stimulation of auricular and body acupuncture materials. *Vet. Acupunc. Newsl.*, Jan.–Mar. 1988, 14(1): 25–36.

Shen, Q.H. and Zheng, K. Treatment of vulvar dystrophy mainly with electro-thermo–AP, *Am. J. Acupunc.*, 1988, 16: 285; ex. CJIT and WM 1988, 8: 27–28.

Shi, H.F. Treatment of 14 cases of flat wart by somatic and auricular acupuncture in combination with cupping. *TCM J. Acupunc. Moxibustion*, 2001, 4(2): 47–49.

Sucks, L.L. Drug addiction: alcoholism, smoking, and obesity treated by auricular staple puncture. *Am. J. Acu.*, 1975, 3(2): 147–150.

Sun, P.H. and Qiao, G.W. Clinical observation of the therapeutic effects of acupuncture combined with auricular plaster therapy on insomnia. *TCM Shang. J. Acupunc. Moxibustion*, 2001, 4(3): 48–49.

Sun, Q.F. and Xu, Y.Q. Obesity treated by auricular acupoint pressure combined with fangfentongsheng pill. Report of 147 cases. *Sichuan Trad. Chin. Med.*, 1988, 6(2): 26–27.

Tan, C.H., Sin, Y.M., and Huang, X.G. The use of laser on acupuncture points for smoking cessation. *Am. J. Acupunc.*, 1987, 15(2): 137–141.

Thoma, H., Benzer, H., Fitzal, S., and Losert, U. On the application of electric currents in operations. Concept of a clinically applicable device. (Author's trans.) *Anaesthesist*, May 1976, 25(5): 239–245, (in German).

Troshin, O.V. A clinico-neurophysiological analysis of the single action of laser puncture. *Like Sprava*, May–Jun. 1994, 5–6: 148–153, (in Russian).

Umeh, B. Ear acupuncture using semi-permanent needles: acceptability, prospects and problems in Nigeria. *Am. J. Acupunc.*, 1988, 16(1–2): 67–70.

Wan, Q. Auricular-plaster therapy plus acupuncture at zusanli for postoperative recovery of intestinal function. *J. Trad. Chin. Med.*, Jun. 2000, 20(2): 134–136.

Wang, W.M. Treatment of 100 cases of pediatric anorexy by burning rush moxibustion. *TCM Shang J. Acupunc. Moxibustion*, 2001, 4(1): 72.

Wen, H.L., Ho, W.K.K., Ling, N. et al. Immunoassayable beta-endorphin level in the plasma and CSF of heroin addicted and normal subjects before and after electroacupuncture. *Am. J. Chin. Med.*, 1980, 8(1–2): 154–159.

Wu, H. et al. Clinical observation and mechanism study in application of auricular-pressing pill for post-operative analgesia. *J. Trad. Chin. Med.*, 1991, 17(1): 26–31.

Xu, R.Z. et al. Observations on the *Curative Effects on Anaphylactic Shock in Mice* by Laser, EAP and *Embedded Needled on Auriculo Acupoints*. Presented at theSecond National Symposium on AP and Moxibustion, Beijing. Foreign Languages Printing House, 1984, p. 147.

Xu, Y. Treatment of acute pain with auricular pellet pressure on ear shenmen as the main point. *J. Trad. Chin. Med.*, Jun. 1992, 12(2): 114–115.

Youbang, C. and Liangyue, D. (Eds.) *Essentials of Contemporary Chinese Acupuncturists' Clinical Experiences.* Foreign Language Press, Beijing, 1989.

Zhang, S.L. Stop smoking with low intensity He–Ne laser. A report of 31 cases. *Jiangxi J. Trad. Chin. Med.*, 1987, 18(4): 39.

Zhang, Q. and Wu, W.Y. Treatment of 193 cases of childhood amblyopia mainly by acupuncture in combination with auricular-plaster therapy. *TCM Shang J. Acupunc. Moxibustion*, 2001, 4(2): 40–42.

Zheng, C.L. Treatment of 58 cases of rheumatoid arthritis by auricular-seed-pressing methods. *TCM Shanghai J. Acupunc. Moxibustion*, 2001, 4(5): 37–38.

Zhu, D. Changes of visual findings, electric findings, electric features and staining of auricles in malignant tumor. *J. Trad. Chin. Med.*, Dec. 1996, 16(4): 247–251.

Zhu, Y., Zhu, B., Yang, Y., Ye, Y., Xu, W., and Wang, P. Reaction of auricular points in rats with experimental gastric ulcer and the action of electro-acupuncture in somatic points. *TCM Shang J. Acupunc. Moxibustion*, 2001, 12(3): 236–241.

Zhu, Y.G., Ye, Y.Y., and Mo, Y.W. The effect of electroacupuncture on the visceral auricular point response in rabbits. *Zhen Ci Yan Jiu*, 1986, 11(3): 234–240, 180, (in Chinese).

chapter seven

Ear diagnosis and morphology

Objectives

- To learn how to perform ear examination and treatment
- To differentiate the characteristics of the normal ear and the unhealthy ear
- To learn the most common general signs of ear pathology
- To learn how to synthesize an ear diagnosis by combining pathology with the points on which it is located
- To learn the most common signs of ear pathology in each organ or body part

Introduction

Because of the reflexive property of the ear, various spontaneous reactions may appear on the auricle when there are disorders of the internal organs or other parts of the body. Such reactions include variations in shape, color, size, and sensation; the appearance of papules, rashes, and discolorations; and increased tenderness or decreased electrical conductivity. Close observation of these changes increases the practitioner's ability to diagnose and treat the patient, both preventatively and concurrently.

Ear diagnosis provides all of the following advantages:

- Allows for the early detection of an illness or disharmony
- Offers a rapid means of the diagnosis of a disorder
- Corroborates the existence of an illness
- Monitors pathological deterioration or improvement of a disorder

Ear diagnosis can be conducted in three ways — through inspection, palpation for tenderness, or through electrical detection.

This chapter emphasizes inspection, which is the primary ear diagnosis method that I use. I palpate for tenderness as a physical way of confirming my diagnosis if it is not corroborated by other methods. I do not use the ear-pressing method through electrical detection. The physician can incorporate ear diagnosis into the physical examination, along with tongue and pulse evaluation, and other methods of diagnosis, as a way of learning more about the patient. (For other books and articles discussing these methods in depth, consult the bibliography at the end of this chapter.)

How to inspect the ear

To interpret abnormal ear findings, one must first have an appreciation of the characteristics of the normal ear and how to systematically examine it. The practitioner may select any of the following as a starting point. You do not need to adhere to this order all of the time because we want to follow the Chinese maxim of treating what we see. Humans, as energetic beings, present differently at different times.

1. Prior to ear diagnosis, do not clean the ear with alcohol as this procedure changes manifestations in the ear. Ear cleansing removes pathological suppurations or scales, or changes the electrical conductivity of the ear. If you see an abnormal color in the ear, it is probably a positive pathological sign. Try to coordinate it with your other diagnostic data. If you are not sure the pathology visible in the ear is accurate, press on the point with the ear probe. If the color does not disappear upon pressure, it is pathological.
2. In performing ear diagnosis, carefully and systematically scan the ear from top to bottom, from medial to lateral, and from front to back. Remember to inspect the back of the ear as well as the underside of the tragus, the antitragus, and the helix. Peruse the ear looking for the most common presentations of ear pathology discussed below. Make a list of your findings on your diagnosis form. As the patient's condition improves or declines, ear pathology changes as well.
3. According to the Law of the Unity of Opposites (*Yin/Yang* theory), conventionally, ear diagnosis is initially performed on the side of the body that corresponds to the patient's gender. Since the right is *Yin* and relates to females, ear diagnosis is performed on a woman's right ear. Since the left is *Yang* and male, ear diagnosis is performed on a male's left ear. However, anatomy is not destiny. Therefore, pay close attention to any anatomical morphology you see in both ears. Such morphology can indicate an existing condition or a constitutional tendency.
4. If the patient complains of pain on a certain side of the body, (i.e., right-sided elbow pain), regardless of gender, inspect the ear on the

same side of the body for pathology (in this case, look at the right ear). However, pathology can appear in the opposite ear. This is due to channel and collateral pathways crossing the body. For instance, because the Large Intestine's divergent meridian emerges from the shoulder at LI 15 and crosses over to the opposite side of the body, right-sided tooth problems may appear in the left ear at the Lower Tooth point. Thus, inspecting the ear on the opposite side of the complaint is an option. Ideally, the practitioner inspects both ears in order to learn as much as possible about the patient.

5. Try to connect the pathology you see with the patient's major complaint, accompanying symptoms, other active complaints, past problems, or family medical history. In virtually every ear there is some pathology, especially in older patients. Data derived from inspection of the ear and the patient interview helps focus one's diagnosis.
6. For example, a diagonal crease in a certain place on the ear lobe is called *Frank's sign* (Figure 7.1). This particular crease indicates heart disease, stress, and high cholesterol. If you see this groove, ask the patient if he or she has any "Heart" pathology. In particular, ask about high cholesterol, stress, and any diagnosed heart problem that he/she may have or that runs in the family. According to classical Oriental theory, such pathology indicates more than the obvious physical heart problems and covers the domain of functions that

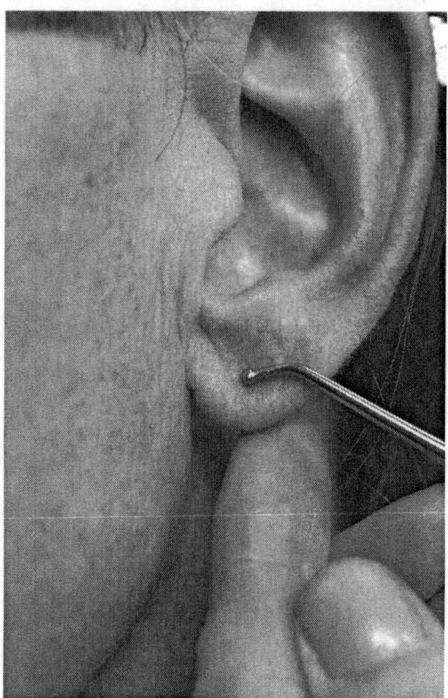

Figure 7.1 Frank's sign.

relate to the Heart in Oriental medicine. Therefore, ask questions such as, "Do you have tightness in the chest, chest pain, palpitations, profuse daytime sweat, chronic persistent cough, insomnia, memory or concentration problems, or emotional problems?" If the patient says "no," check his or her pulse, tongue, and complexion, which also may indicate Heart conditions. If the patient still does not make an affirmative answer, inquire about any family history of heart problems. The patient may have a genetic predisposition to heart problems, even though bodily signs and symptoms have not yet developed. Thus, the ear can be a valuable tool in revealing constitutional predispositions.

7. At first, patients might answer your questions in the negative. However, probe more deeply. Patients frequently report back at a later time that after having thought about your questions they do indeed have some of these conditions. These disorders simply were not at the top of the patient's list of complaints at the time of questioning.

The characteristics of the normal ear

1. Normal ears should be similar in size and placement to each other, and should move freely and painlessly when massaged. Ideally, the normal ear is firm but flexible, not too soft, not too thick or too hard. Prominent and pendulous ears in the elderly are a sign of atrophy and aging, and normal for that age group.
2. The auricles should be free of scales, redness, and inflammation, have normal moisture, be clean, and of the same color as the rest of the skin on the body. The helix should have a reddish hue. As mentioned earlier, according to Oriental medicine, the ear is related to the Kidney. Scholar Manfred Porkert states, "Thus it is the outward appearance of the ear that may orient us on the state of the constitutive, unborn energies deposited in the *o. renalis* (kidney). The ear conch should be moderately fleshy, with a subdued luster that indicates sufficient *Qi nativum* (congenital *Qi*)."[1] Hence, the condition of the ear tells us about the health of the Kidney, the root *Qi* of the body, and the basis of immunity.
3. Prior to ear treatment, clean it with 70% alcohol. Normal earwax or dirt will be removed easily; otherwise, the deposit may be pathological.

The abnormal ear: ear pathology and its clinical differentiation

Many illnesses have as a defining characteristic an abnormal presentation in the external auricle. This should not be surprising since the ear reflects the condition of the entire body. Manifestations of pathology in the ear include the following characteristics.

- Asymmetries
- Abnormal color including erythema, flushing, paleness, bluish-black coloration
- Excess moisture or oozing rash
- Abnormal hair growth
- Birthmarks
- Engorged blood vessels and abnormal blood color (blue, red, or purple)
- Dilated capillaries, varicosities, hyperpigmentation, and capillary clustering
- Boils, blisters, warts, lesions, moles, papules, pimples
- Bruises
- Dark spots, petechiae
- Depressions, grooves, creases, such as Frank's sign
- Swelling, edema, puffiness, bloating
- Prolapses
- Dry, scaly, leathery, withered skin, skin abrasions, erosions, skin breakdown, desquamation
- Detached ear lobes, ears that move, high ears, ears that stick out, small ears, long ears lying close to the head
- Pathology of the helix, conchas, or antihelix crus
- Red veins on the posterior aspect of the ears
- Hard nodules or calculi on the rim of the auricle or on the outside opening of the external auditory meatus
- Fleshy, scaly, painful, crusty lesions
- Knots, lumps, bumps, growths, protuberant stripes, ridges
- Scars
- Shiny spots
- Shriveled, shrunken ears

The most common signs of point pathology that I have gleaned from my clinical experience are summarized in Table 7.1. Part One of the chart offers general pathology and Part Two is more specific. To use this chart effectively for diagnosis, combine the pathology (i.e., redness) with the point on which it is found (i.e., Lungs) to construct the proper diagnosis, which would be Heat in the Lungs. This simple process of combining the abnormal finding with the point on the ear promotes rapid and accurate diagnosis and the reasoning process over memorization so that one is free from memorizing and/or having to consult written lists of pathology. Thus, the practitioner learns to quickly infer the clinical differentiation presented in the ear.

For instance, red signifies Heat and Heat Stasis. Let us say you see a red mark on the Stomach area. This suggests the broad category of Heat or Heat Stasis in the Stomach, which can have multiple manifestations, such as a Stomach ulcer, excess hunger and thirst, bad breath, or acid reflux disease. Specifically, we should not equate Heat in the Stomach with an ulcer or any other Western illness because, as Oriental medical physicians, we differen-

Table 7.1 Clinical Differentiation of Ear Pathology

Finding	Differentiation
Part One	
Asymmetrical shape	Evaluate pathology in body in relation to where pathology appears in the ear
Abnormal color, including erythema, flushing, paleness, bluish-black coloration	Heat, Heat Stasis, inflammatory disease, Cold Stagnation, deficiency, *Qi* Stagnation, Blood Stagnation
Excessive moisture or oozing rash; red and oozing	Excess Dampness, Damp-Heat
Abnormal hair growth	Hormonal problems, Kidney *Qi* deficiency
Birthmarks	Blood Stagnation
Engorged blood vessels and abnormal blood color (blue, red, or purple)	Circulatory problems
Dilated capillaries, varicosities, hyperpigmentation, and capillary clustering	Circulatory problems, Cold Stagnation, Heat Stasis, *Qi,* and/or Blood Stagnation, extravasation
Boils, blisters, warts, lesions, moles, papules, and pimples	Damp-Heat, Toxic-Heat, Heat, Dampness, or Fire
Bruises	Blood Stagnation and/or extravasations, trauma
Dark spots, petechiae	Stagnant Blood, Heat Stasis, Blood Stasis
Depressions, grooves, and creases (such as Frank's sign)	Deficiency in corresponding area; risk of heart attack, high cholesterol, coronary artery disease, stress, and anxiety
Swelling, edema, puffiness, bloating	Damp, Water, Dilute Phlegm, Phlegm, *Yang* deficiency
Prolapses	Deficiency of area
Dry, scaly, leathery, withered skin; skin abrasions, erosions, skin breakdown, desquamation	Psoriasis or seborrhea, Blood deficiency, *Yin* deficiency, *Yang* deficiency, poor absorption, or dermal disease
Ears that move and are positioned high on the head	Eats excess animal food
Ears that stick out	*Yin* constitution, poor hearing, narrow viewpoint (see Kushi[3])
Detached ear lobes	Eats more vegetable food
Long ears lying close to head	Balanced, makes sound judgments
Long ear lobe (ear lobe length equals one third the length of the entire ear)	
Small ears	Limited perspective
Pathology of the helix	Circulatory system problems
Pathology of the inner ear (conchas)	Digestive system problems
Pathology of the middle ear (antihelix crus)	Nervous system problems

Table 7.1 (continued) Clinical Differentiation of Ear Pathology

Finding	Differentiation
Red veins on the posterior aspect of cold ears	Precursor to measles or small pox: medium red = slight infection, purple = average infection, bluish-black = serious small pox infection
Hard nodules or calculi on rim of auricle or on the outside of the external auditory meatus	Phlegm
Fleshy, scaly, painful, crusty lesions	Refer to physician
Knots, lumps, bumps, growths, protuberant stripes, or ridges	*Qi* Stagnation, Blood Stagnation, Damp, Phlegm, desiccated feces
Scars	Potential organ/meridian disturbances, organ removal
Shiny spots	Organ removal
Shriveled, shrunken ear	Decline of *Qi* and overall weakness
Part Two	
Red dots at the end of Stomach area (round area); more underneath the crus	Gastric ulcer, acid reflux disease
Red end of the crus to round area above the Stomach point	Duodenal ulcer
Faded dot to curvature above the crus	Past history of duodenal ulcer
Lumps, protrusions in the Stomach area	Chronic gastritis
Lumps, protrusions in the Gallbladder area	Chronic cholelithiasis
Lumps, protrusions in the Pancreas area	Chronic pancreatitis
Lumps, protrusions in Large Intestine area	Chronic constipation
Lumps, protrusions in the Liver area	Fatty liver
Depression in Low Blood Pressure point	Hypotension
Groove from Low Blood Pressure point to Neurasthenia point	Hypotension
Clusters of nodules	Tumors/cancer
Protrusion in Occiput point	Occipital headache
Protrusion in Temple point	Temporal headache
Protrusion in Forehead point	Frontal headache
Protrusion in Neck area	Cervical disease
Capillaries at Ankle point	Injury of ankle joint
Swelling at Hemorrhoid point	Hemorrhoids
Flaky, desquamation in triangular fossa at Uterus point	Leukorrhea
Red triangular fossa	Menstruation
Tinnitus groove	Tinnitus
Firm ear	Strong Kidney function

(*continued*)

Table 7.1 (continued) Clinical Differentiation of Ear Pathology

Finding	Differentiation
Thinner and softer ear	Weak Kidney function
Yellow, black, blue helix	Poor prognosis
Thin white/thin black ear	Disturbance of Kidneys
Withered helix with a layer of dust	Bone disorder
Dried-up helix	Diabetes
Fused helix with scapha	Congenital fusion
Dual Darwin's tubercle	Normal
Missing Darwin's tubercle	Weak immunity
Red in scapha	Dermatitis

tiate the syndrome (i.e., Heat/Heat Stasis in the Stomach) rather than diagnose an illness (i.e., Stomach ulcer). There are many possible health disorders that are covered under the proper differentiation of the syndrome vs. any one particular disease. This is a unique strength of Oriental medicine, which treats the syndrome pattern.

In another case, if the red mark is found on a Throat point, the diagnosis is Heat in the throat. Heat here could take the form of a sore throat in its many varieties.

The Nanking Army Ear Acupuncture Book and other texts found in the reference section of this chapter provide complex lists correlating pathology with auriculoacupoints. They can be consulted for additional specific clinical information.

Ear pathology

- **Asymmetries** — as we have seen, both ears should be symmetrical in shape, and similar in size, color, and moisture. Compare the right and left auricles in relation to the pathologies listed above and evaluate the differences. In particular, note the location of these pathologies. Injury may account for some variation, so inquire about any injuries if there are gross differences between the two ears. Pathological changes can differ from ear to ear because pathology tends to occur in the same ear as on the affected side of the body or on the side corresponding to gender. Generally speaking, if the pathology is found on both ears, the pathology is more chronic.
- **Abnormal color includes erythema, flushing, paleness, bluish-black coloration** — erythema or redness is common in the ear. Red areas or marks can occur. Redness indicates Heat, Heat Stasis, or inflammatory disease. Consider the redness carefully by interpreting the Heat in relation to where the redness is found. For instance, a red mark on the Hemorrhoid point may indicate hemorrhoids due to Stagnant Blood with Heat or a red mark on the Common Cold

point may mean a Wind–Heat invasion. Flushing colorations can be interpreted like red marks. Rashes are also interpreted this way. If red, the rash means Heat in the Blood or Heat leading to Blood Stasis. Paleness indicates Deficiency of the affected area. Bluish-black colorations are indicative of Cold Stagnation. Pale purple suggests *Qi* Stagnation and reddish purple signifies Blood Stagnation.

- **Excess moisture or oozing rash** — both of these findings indicate excess Dampness in the body. If the rash is red and oozing, Damp-Heat is the diagnosis.
- **Abnormal hair growth** — as men age, hair may be found in the auricle. This is a sign of hormonal changes that accompany the decline of Kidney *Qi*, which occurs with aging. Thus, the amount of hair in the auricle gives us an idea as to the state of the person's Kidney *Qi*.
- **Birthmarks** — birthmarks can range in color from purple to blue, black, red, or faded brown. They are generally viewed as signs and symptoms of Stagnant Blood. Note where the birthmark is on the ear and then see if the patient has any Blood Stagnation in the corresponding area or organ of the body.
- **Engorged blood vessels and abnormal blood color (blue, red, or purple)** — inspect the ear for visible blood vessels. In addition to looking at the ear for the location of this sign, also consider the color of the blood within the vessel. Color differentiation can further assist you with understanding etiology and directing treatment. Blue blood in the vessel indicates Stagnation due to Cold. Heavy pain in the body corresponding to the area of the vessel on the auricle is another further indication of Blood Stagnation due to Cold. Red denotes Heat and/or Heat Stasis. Pale purple is *Qi* Stagnation and reddish purple is Blood Stagnation with Heat.
- **Dilated capillaries, varicosities, hyperpigmentation, and capillary clustering** — dilated capillaries or varicosities (blood engorged vessels or blood extravasations) on the ear indicate circulatory problems elsewhere in the body, such as varicose veins in the legs or insufficiency of circulation to body parts such as the hips. The Knee and Ankle points commonly exhibit capillary clustering. Hyperpigmentation and capillary clustering, which are also signs of Blood Stagnation, can be seen if there are old, unresolved lesions.
- **Boils, blisters, warts, lesions, moles, papules, and pimples** — boils or blisters indicate Damp-Heat or Toxic Heat in the body. Interpret the location of Toxic Heat by examining the area on the ear where the boil develops. If papules and pimples are red, they indicate Heat; if white, Dampness. Red moles and reddish pink warts also point to Heat in the Blood. If the mole is brown or black (a stronger form of Heat), Fire is present.
- **Bruises** — bruises, indicative of Blood Stagnation or Blood extravasations, do not develop spontaneously on the ear. If bruises are

present, they are caused either from ear therapies or from other external sources, such as trauma to the ear. However, the ear will not bruise with the proper application of ear modalities. If bruising does occur, check that you and your patient are applying the modalities appropriately.

- **Dark spots, petichiae** — dark spots (vs. a bruise) can develop on the ear. They also indicate Stagnation. The patient may have pain in the area of the body corresponding to the dark spot. Petechiae are small dots that are generally red or purple. Petechiae indicate Heat Stasis (if red) or Blood Stasis (if reddish purple).
- **Depressions, grooves, and creases, such as Frank's sign** — depressions and small pore-like structures found on points that are not inherently concave indicate deficiency in the corresponding body part or organ. For instance, if the Spleen area tends to be depressed, Spleen *Qi* Deficiency is indicated. The Lung and Heart points frequently are depressed indicating Lung *Qi* deficiency in the former and Heart *Qi* deficiency in the latter case.

  Frank's sign was first reported in 1973 by pulmonologist Saunders Frank. Romoli et al.[2] remind us that "Frank's sign, a diagonal crease on the earlobe, is detectable especially after the age of 40. This is commonly accepted as a sign of coronary heart disease even in Western medicine."

  The crease extends from the Lower Blood Pressure point laterally on a diagonal (see Figure 7.1). A person with Frank's sign is significantly more likely (eight times more likely) to die from heart disease than a person without such a crease. Those with a crease and established heart disease are three times more likely to die from heart disease as those with established heart disease and no crease. Most studies link Frank's sign with high cholesterol as the precipitating factor in heart disease. Some authors report an association between anxiety and coronary heart disease. Romoli et al.[2] write, "Our work group of 143 patients with ear lobe creases showed — in both sexes and in all examined decades (fifth, sixth, and seventh) — higher levels of anxiety than in the control group."

  Like all ear pathologies, Frank's sign can retreat if the person's health improves. If the fissure on the lobe heals, according to Kushi,[3] then the person is eating a macrobiotic diet (i.e., no animal fat, which helps reduce high cholesterol and coronary artery disease).
- **Swelling, edema, puffiness, bloating** — in contrast to depressions, swelling, edema, puffiness, and bloating signify Damp, Water, Dilute Phlegm, Phlegm, or *Yang* Deficiency.
- **Prolapses** — prolapses are different from depressions or indentations. A prolapse appears on an ear structure as a "collapsed" part or border. Interpret the prolapse as a more pronounced deficiency, called in Oriental medicine "collapse of the *Qi* or *Yang*" in the corre-

sponding area. Common places where prolapses occur are in the Spleen point, the Spinal Vertebrae points, and the Antitragus area.

When a prolapse occurs in the Spleen area, the lateral border of the Spleen point is not firm and intact. This indicates Spleen *Yang* deficiency or a Collapse of Spleen *Qi*. When seen along the spinal portion of the ear, the antihelix crus lacks a clear, firm border, indicating a vertebral problem, such as herniated disks. The prolapsed Antitragus area results in a turned down antitragus instead of an antitragus oriented firmly upward, as in the case of the smart crest (Figure 7.2 and Figure 7.3). The prolapsed antitragus is seen in cases of weakness and exhaustion.

- **Dry, scaly, leathery, withered skin; skin abrasions, erosions, breakdown, desquamation** — dry skin (or leathery, withered skin) is a common finding in the ear. Such presentations (from a Chinese viewpoint) indicate *Yin* or Blood deficiency. *Yang* deficiency is also a possibility. In that case, the *Yang* is failing to generate the fluids and the Blood. In Western medicine, dry skin may present as psoriasis, dermatitis, or seborrhea. Note the points where the dryness is found. Skin breakdowns, abrasions, erosions, and desquamation can be caused from reclining excessively on that ear. The problem is also related to poor absorption or can be related to other dermatological diseases.

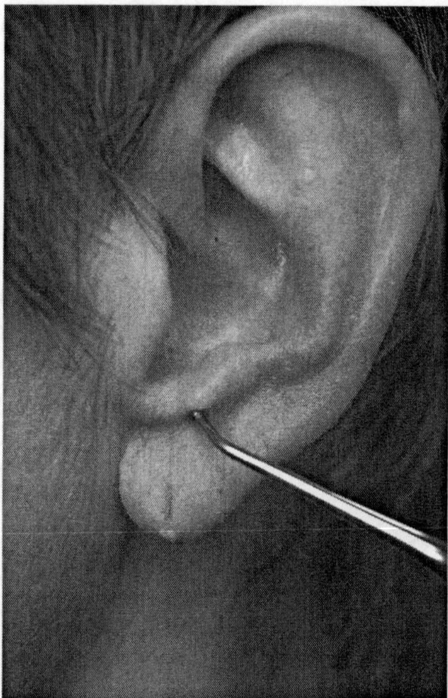

Figure 7.2 A partially prolapsed antitragus.

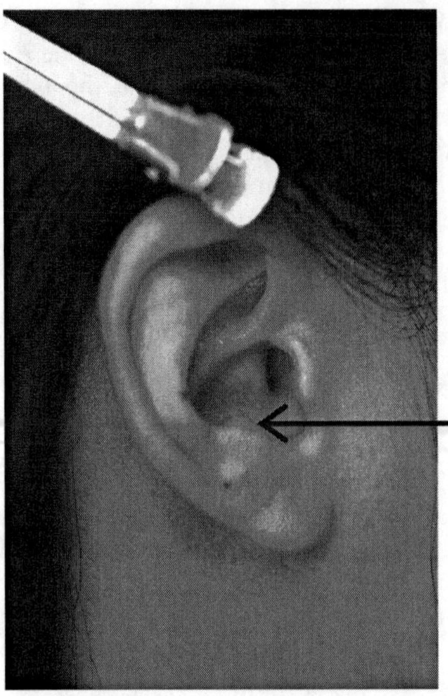

Figure 7.3 The smart crest.

- **Ears that move and are positioned high on the head, ears that stick out, detached ear lobes, long ears lying close to the head, small ears** — Michio Kushi[3] maintains that "ears that move on the head and are positioned high on the head indicate that the person eats an excess of animal food, and ears that stick out mean that the person has a *Yin* constitution." Because of this feature, Kushi writes, "Physiologically, hearing tends to be poor." The ears of many elderly present this way. Mentally, he says such people tend to have a narrow point of view. "Ears that are detached mean that the person eats more vegetarian food. Kushi continues, "Long ears lying close to the head mean that the person makes sound judgements and small ears mean that the person has a limited perspective." Kushi changed some *Yin/Yang* theory so consult his book to understand this concept.
- **Pathology of the helix, conchas, or antihelix crus** — Kushi[3] attributes circulatory disorders to pathology found on the helix. "Problems on the conchas suggest digestive problems. Problems of the middle ear (that is, the antihelix crus) suggest nervous system problems."
- **Red veins on the posterior aspect of the ears** — Manfred Porkert[4] says "If there are red veins on the posterior aspect of the ears and the ears are cold, this is a precursor to measles or small pox. Medium red color indicates slight infection, purple is average infection, and bluish-black signifies a serious small pox infection."

- **Hard nodules or calculi on the rim of the auricle or on the outside opening of the external auditory meatus** — phlegm accumulations are commonly seen in the ear, especially in the Constipation area and in the Stomach. A phlegm ridge in the Constipation area is indicative of fecal accumulation or constipation. Phlegm accumulations are frequently seen in the Stomach area of the auricle. Remember, the Stomach point extends halfway across the width of the cavum concha. Because Phlegm can accumulate within the Stomach and, hence, appear on the Stomach ear point, the end of the crus of the helix will seem longer than usual, thus making the Stomach point look as though it extends farther across the concha. However, the crus is not longer. It is the presence of Phlegm in the Stomach that gives this impression. I have termed this particular morphology the *Phlegm ridge*.

  To correctly locate the Stomach point, try the following technique: put your ear probe on the crus of the helix and slide off of the crus with the probe laterally until you fall into a small depression. This is the end of the crus and, therefore, the beginning of the Stomach point. Then, extend the lateral border of the Stomach point halfway across the concha, and you have located the lateral border of the Stomach point.
- **Fleshy, scaly, painful, crusty lesions** — any ear mark that has color variations to it, or any ear growth should be considered suspicious and examined by a dermatologist to ensure that the lesions are not cancerous or precancerous. If the lesions are cancerous, there may be local swelling of the lymph nodes. However, this possible cancerous condition is not for the acupuncturist to evaluate or diagnose. The ear is susceptible to skin cancer since it is so exposed to the environment and may not have received adequate sun protection. Instruct your patients to avoid unprotected sun exposure.
- **Knots, lumps, bumps, growths, protuberant stripes, or ridges** — knots, lumps, bumps, growths, protuberant stripes, or ridges can indicate *Qi* Stagnation, Blood Stagnation, or the presence of Dampness, Phlegm, or desiccated feces. If white or hard in nature, knots or bumps can be due to uric acid crystals, or Damp or Phlegm accumulations. A white, hard, long, even, bony phlegm ridge can indicate long-term constipation, whereas if the area has a soft white center, the bowel movement may be sluggish. Such lumps can also indicate arthritis and are frequently seen in the Neck and Cervical vertebrae area or on the rim of the helix. Purple lumps sometimes appear on the Uterus point and indicate uterine fibroid tumors.

  Once you learn how to differentiate these pathologies you can safely treat the underlying disorder that causes their development. However, if you are unsure as to the nature of the growth, refer the patient to a dermatologist for proper evaluation and treatment.

- **Scars** — scars on the ear caused by external factors, such as injury to the ear, may produce energy disruption in the corresponding body areas. Likewise, injury to a body part or organ removal may appear as a small crescent-shape scar in the ear.
- **Shiny spots** — shiny spots often develop on the ear in the identical place where an organ was surgically removed.
- **Shriveled, shrunken ears** — shriveled, shrunken ears indicate the decline of *Qi* and overall weakness.

Organ, body system, and body part pathology

Apart from the general pathological categories discussed above, specific pathology relating to organs, body systems, or body parts can now be understood. This information is organized into diagnostic categories so that the practitioner can see the most common pathology within each category, its clinical meanings, and the logical sense that they make in relation to a diagnosis. Corresponding photos are presented with the discussion. Studying the photos along with the information in this chapter assists the practitioner at becoming visually adept at recognizing and diagnosing these pathologies.

Respiratory disorders

Depressions

Respiratory disorders in the ear usually show up in the form of two pathologies — depressions or red marks. A depression is one that is deeper than the size of the normal point depth. Some depressions are very deep and some appear like several enlarged pores.

Depressions indicate deficiency of the point on which it is found. Depressions on the Lung points, which are the points pertaining to the major respiratory organ, indicate Lung *Qi* deficiency. Lung *Qi* deficiency manifests as asthma, shortness of breath, fatigue and allergies, tightness in the chest, and even walking pneumonia. Figure 7.4 to Figure 7.6 illustrate depressions on the Lung points.

Heat shows up as redness on the body. Heat on the Allergy point indicates allergies that have Heat characteristics, such as nasal congestion, yellow mucus, low-grade fever, slight sore throat, red tongue, thin yellow coat, and slightly fast superficial pulse. The allergies may be respiratory allergies or skin allergies, such as rashes or pimples, since the Lungs dominate the skin (Figure 7.7).

Cardiovascular problems

Depressions

Cardiovascular problems show up in the ear in several places. Depressions and grooves are indicative of deficiency. As shown in Figure 7.8, depressions

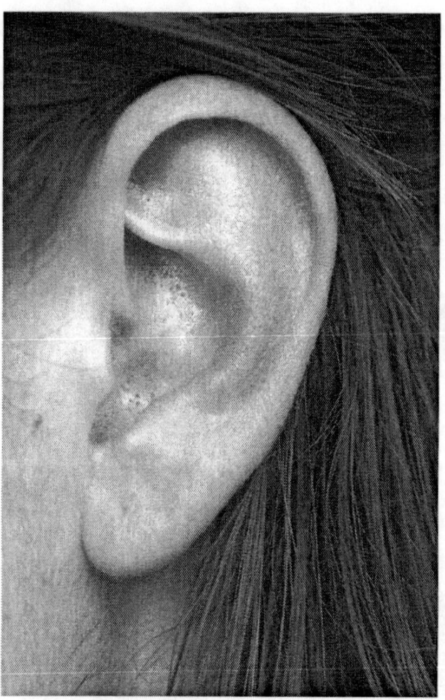

Figure 7.4 Small pore-like depressions on the Upper and Lower Lung points (patient has shortness of breath and tightness in the chest, accompanying walking pneumonia).

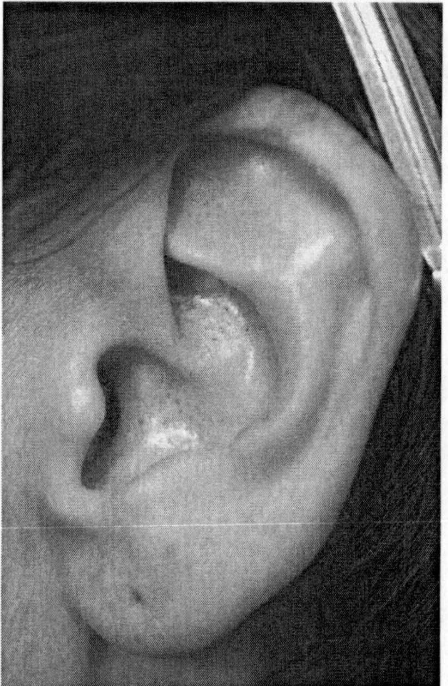

Figure 7.5 Small pore-like depressions on the Upper and Lower Lung points as well as the deep Heart point (patient has fatigue and shortness of breath).

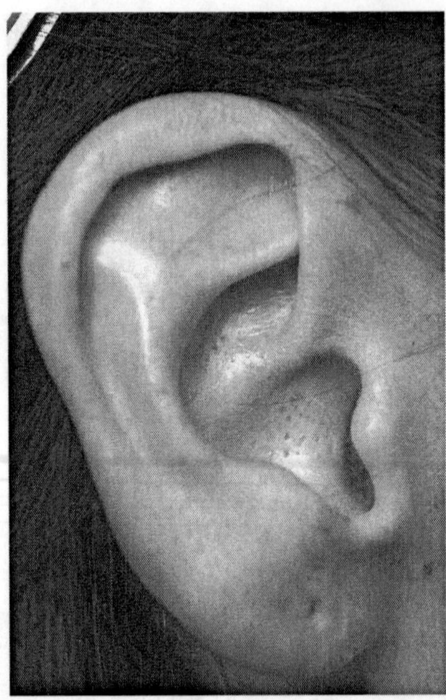

Figure 7.6 Small pore-like depressions on the Upper and Lower Lung points as well as on the Heart point (patient has shortness of breath in the morning).

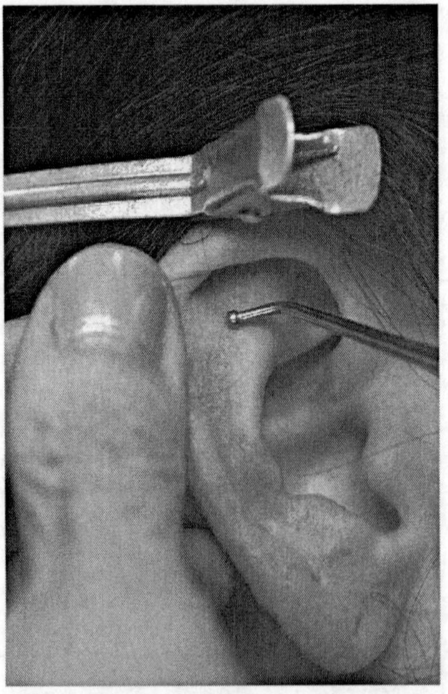

Figure 7.7 Redness in the scapha on the Allergy point (patient has allergies and dermatitis; red appearing on this point [not visible in this black and white photo] has the clinical differentiation of allergies).

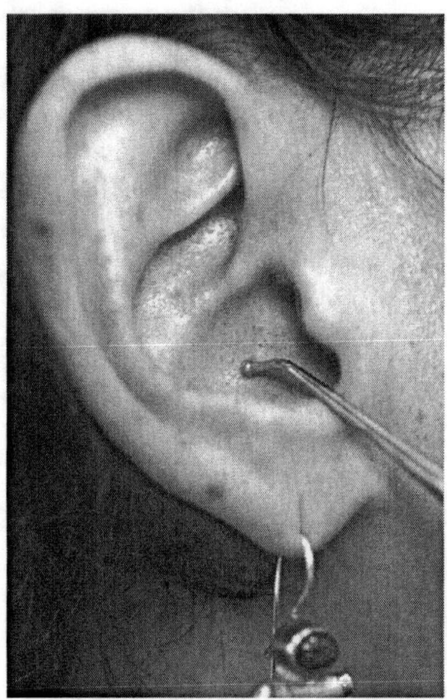

Figure 7.8 A deep, depressed Heart point (patient has palpitations, a tendency to worry, tingling feeling in the hands at night, tightness in the mid-back and chest, low blood pressure, a heart murmur, and received three blood transfusions at birth due to an Rh incompatibility).

in the Heart area indicates Heart *Qi* deficiency. Clinical manifestations of Heart *Qi* deficiency include high blood pressure, a family history of heart disease, and shortness of breath, palpitations, low blood pressure, numbness and tingling in the arms and hands, and more.

Grooves

The low blood pressure groove suggests heart pathology as well, and originates from the Low Blood Pressure point (Figure 7.9). The low blood pressure groove does not travel on an angle like Frank's sign, but rather folds vertically downward, resembling a collapsed fold in the skin.

Frank's sign, as we have seen earlier in this chapter, is a diagonal crease on the ear lobe that originates in the lower blood pressure area and extends downward on a diagonal line laterally across the lobe. In general, the longer the crease and deeper the crease, the more serious and long-term the problem is. Compare the difference between the low blood pressure groove and Frank's sign (see Figure 7.1).

Redness

Red indicates heat. A red Heart point indicates heat in the Heart, which produces restlessness and insomnia, or other Chinese "Heat in the Heart problems (Figure 7.10). (Unfortunately, the color pathology cannot be depicted

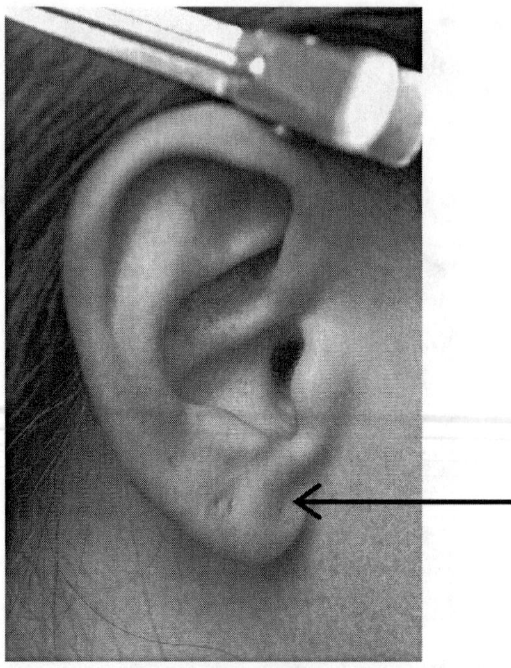

Figure 7.9 The low blood pressure groove (patient has low blood pressure).

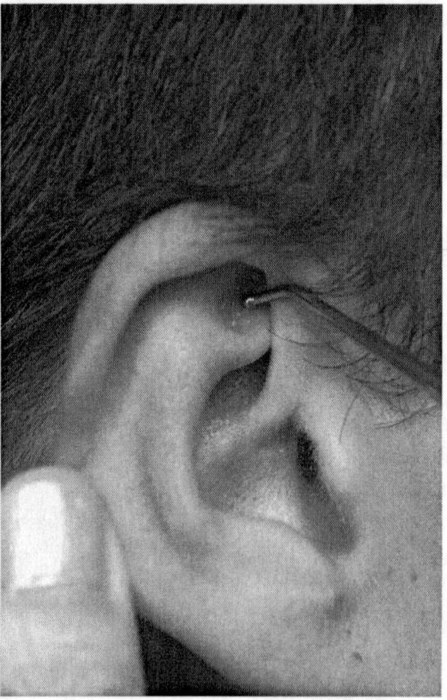

Figure 7.10 Suppuration at *Shenmen* (patient has anxiety, skin rashes, and nausea).

in the black and white photos.) Heat may cause rashes and oozing of fluids at the Heart point or points related to the Heart, most notably *Shenmen*.

Hepatobiliary/gastrointestinal problems (stomach, spleen, liver, gallbladder, and small intestine)

Several organs are part of the hepatobiliary/gastrointestinal systems and many illnesses fall within their domain. The most common clinical pathologies found in the ear pertaining to these systems are discussed and shown below.

Phlegm ridge

The phlegm ridge is a frequently observed formation in the ear, specifically the phlegm ridge in the Stomach area. The phlegm ridge indicates that Dampness or Phlegm are being retained in the stomach either due to weak Stomach *Qi* failing to rotten and ripen the food, or Phlegm created through consumption of the proper *Yin* of the Stomach by Heat or Liver *Qi* stagnation. Phlegm in the Stomach can cause many symptoms, including nausea, stomach pain, food stagnation symptoms, and abdominal distention (Figure 7.11 and Figure 7.12).

Puffiness

Puffiness of specific organ points in the gastrointestinal/hepatobiliary systems is frequently seen in the ear. The Spleen area typically appears as puffy,

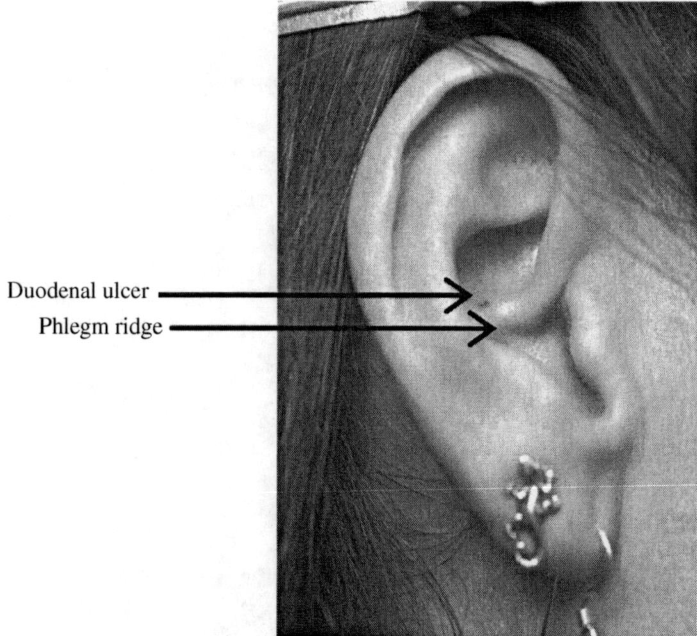

Figure 7.11 Phlegm ridge and duodenal ulcer (patient has knotted abdominal pain precisely at the center of the Stomach [CV 12, *Zhongwan*]).

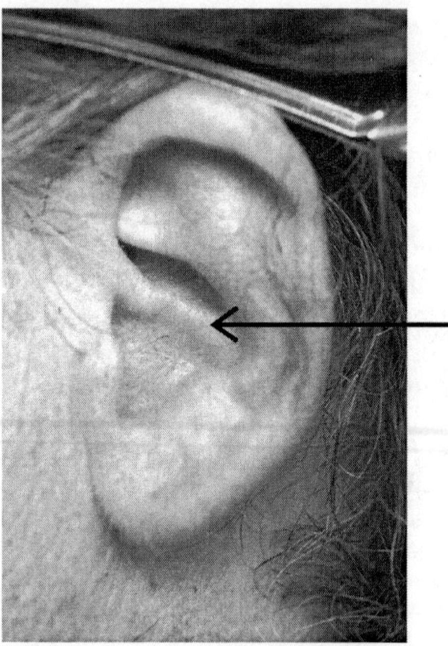

Figure 7.12 Long phlegm ridge extending to the Spleen area (patient experiences Stomach pain, Liver pain, fatigue, pallor, loose stools, abdominal distention and gas, signs and symptoms of Spleen *Qi* deficiency).

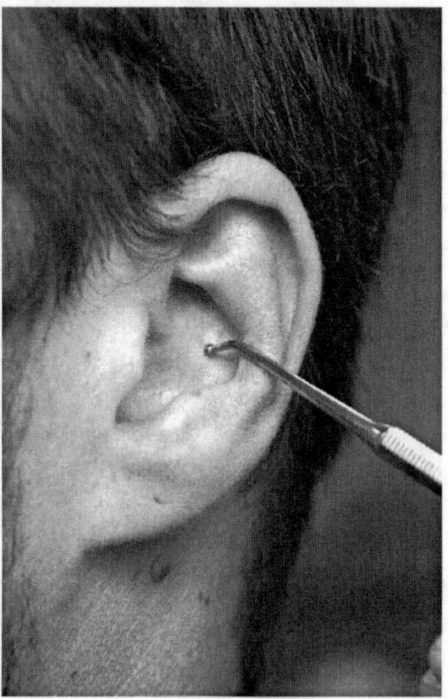

Figure 7.13 Puffy Stomach and Spleen points (patient experiences nausea caused by Damp retention in the Spleen and Stomach).

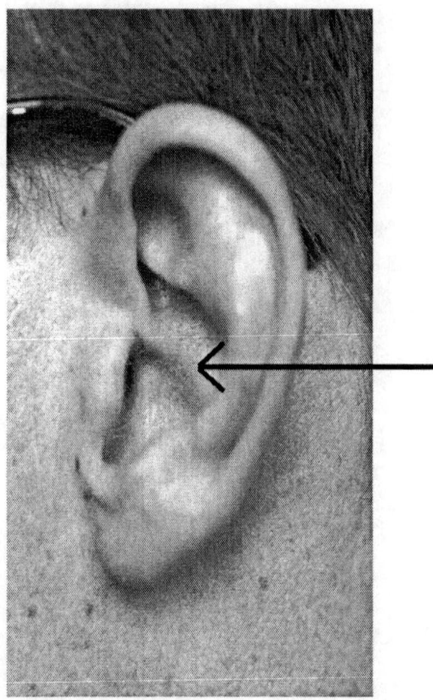

Figure 7.14 Puffy Spleen point (patient has abdominal distention as a major complaint; a cardinal symptom of Spleen *Qi* deficiency).

a clear example of Spleen *Qi* Deficiency where the Spleen fails to transform and transport the digestate, which results in Damp retention or puffiness (Figure 7.13 and Figure 7.14).

Red marks

Heat in the Stomach and Liver areas is a common clinical finding. Heat shows up as redness, while ulcers with heat manifestations show up as red marks. Figure 7.11 also illustrates a duodenal ulcer. Note the dark spot at the end of the Stomach point and the beginning of the Duodenum point. This patient has a duodenal ulcer, experiences what she describes as knotted abdominal pain, and reports a high level of stress, a leading cause of ulcers.

Collapsed borders

The Spleen tends toward deficiency and Collapse of *Yang*. This syndrome shows up as a collapsed Spleen border (Figure 7.15).

Stagnation is typified by its characteristic purple color. Purple in the Liver area indicates Liver pain and on the Pancreas suggests pancreas disorders, such as hypoglycemia.

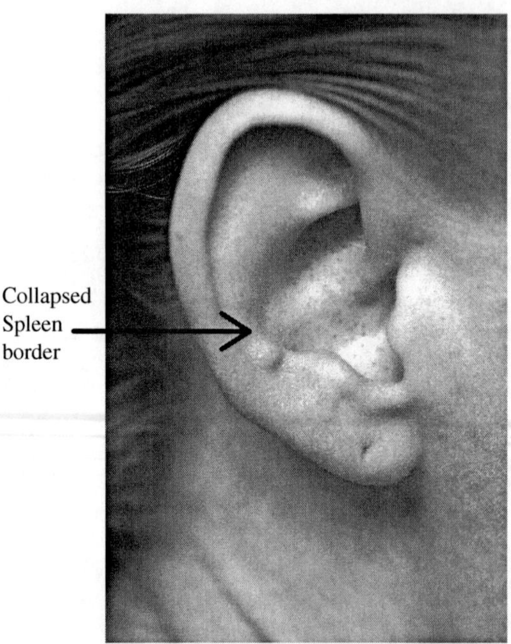

Figure 7.15 Collapsed Spleen border and large bump in the Upper Thoracic/Lower Cervical areas (patient has all the common signs and symptoms of Spleen *Qi* deficiency).

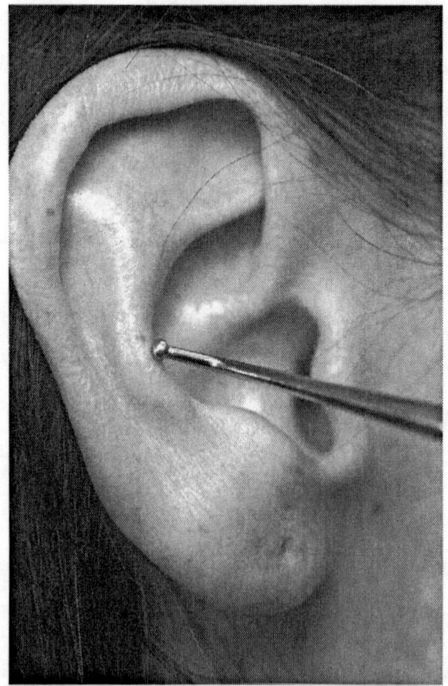

Figure 7.16 Brown dot on Mammary points (indicates old Blood Stagnation in the breast such as occurs in fibrocystic breasts).

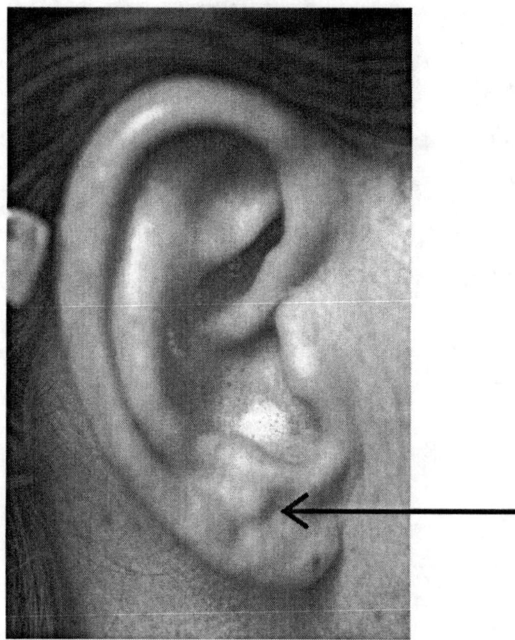

Figure 7.17 Puffy Forehead point (patient has sinus infection).

Organ pathologies and diseases

Miscellaneous organ pathologies appear in the ear as well. Some of them are representatively included here (Figure 7.16 to Figure 7.18).

Eye, ear, nose, and throat pathology

The Eye groove, sometimes referred to as the Myopia groove, forms a crease or fold originating from the Eye 1 point and travels downward. It consistently indicates problems with vision, especially nearsightedness (Figure 7.19). Some hearing problems such as tinnitus (ear ringing) also appear in the ear as a groove called the Tinnitus groove (Figure 7.20).

Scars

If not caused by direct injury, scars in the ear represent removal of an organ or body part. Marks can be viewed similarly to scars and indicate problems on the point where they are found (Figure 7.21 and Figure 7.22).

Musculoskeletal disorders

Capillaries

Capillaries are indicative of circulation problems, trauma, or surgeries. They are commonly seen in the ear, particularly in the lower extremities, such as the hip, knees, and ankles, which tend towards poor circulation (Figure 7.23).

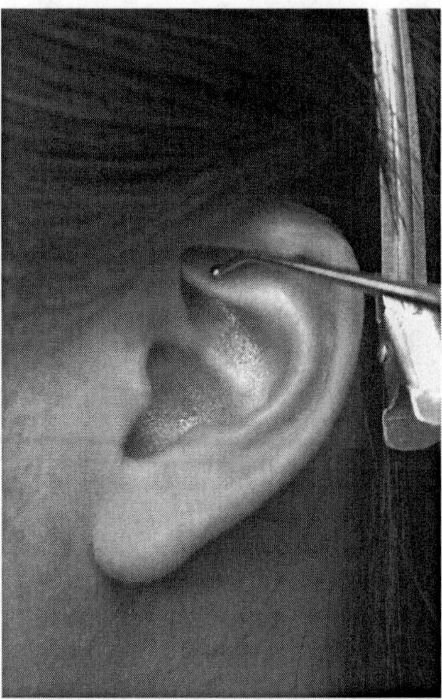

Figure 7.18 Constipation ridge (patient has long-term constipation).

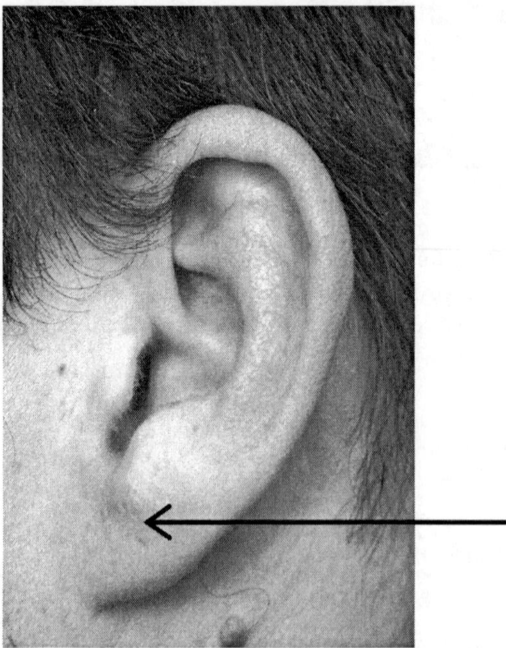

Figure 7.19 Myopia groove (patient is nearsighted, has floaters, decreased nighttime vision, frequent red eyes, and skin patches around the eyes).

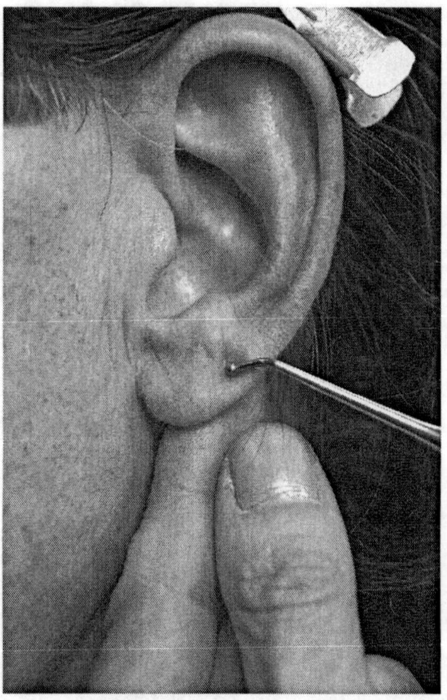

Figure 7.20 Tinnitus groove (patient has ringing in the ears and vision problems).

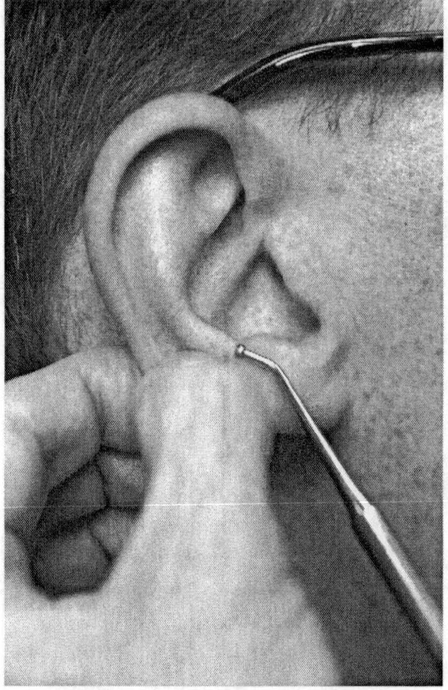

Figure 7.21 Mark on the Throat point (patient has had a tonsillectomy).

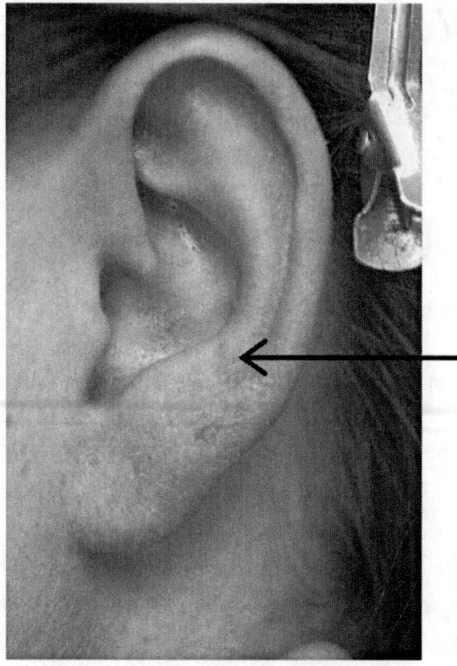

***Figure** 7.22* Scar on the Throat point (patient has had a tonsillectomy).

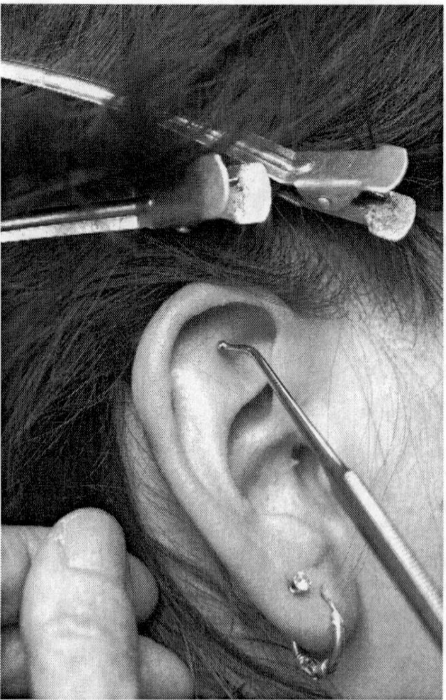

***Figure** 7.23* Capillaries in the Ankle area (patient has weak ankles).

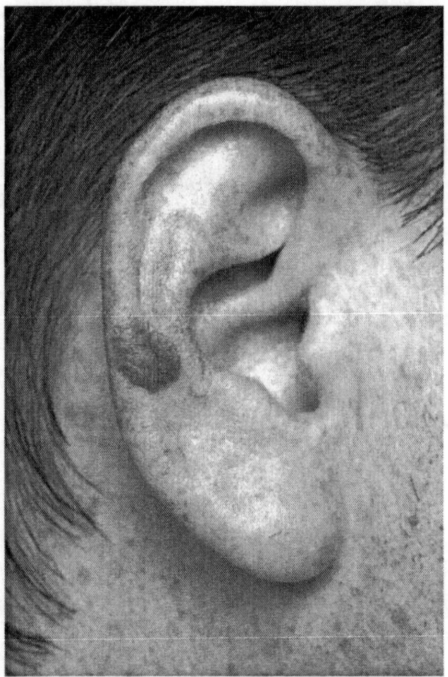

Figure 7.24 Birthmark on the Shoulder area (congential shoulder weakness).

As discussed earlier in this chapter, birthmarks are viewed as Blood Stagnation, which may affect the areas on which they are found (Figure 7.24).

Neck pathology

Bumps, lumps, ridges, and arthritic bone growths

Structurally bumps, lumps, ridges, and arthritic bone growths are very similar as are their diagnostic meanings. Essentially these structures can be viewed as Excesses. They are the opposite of grooves or depressions that are caused by deficiencies (Figure 7.25 to Figure 7.27).

Congenital morphology

Two examples of a high, pronounced antitragus (also called a smart crest), which indicates high intelligence, are shown here (Figure 7.28; also see Figure 7.3). A deviation of the antihelix crus and a ridge in the cymba concha are also congenital.

Miscellaneous pathology

A pathological lumpy ear is a good ear to benefit from massage (Figure 7.29).

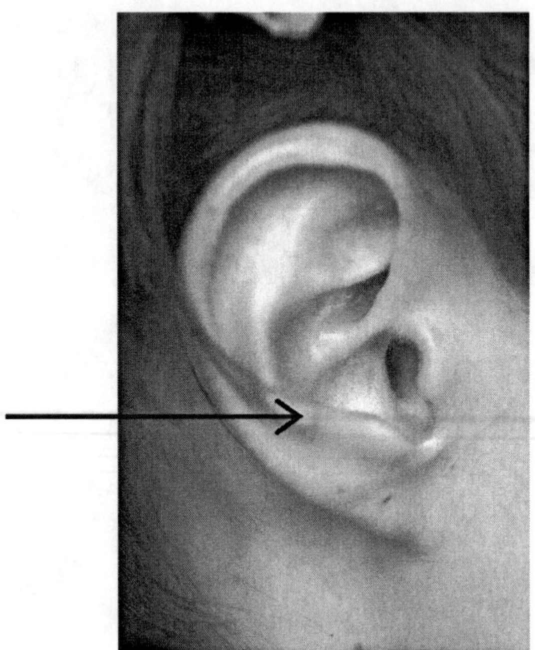

Figure 7.25 White bump on the Neck area (patient had cervical disease [see another large bump in the Upper Thoracic/Lower Cervical areas in Figure 7.15]).

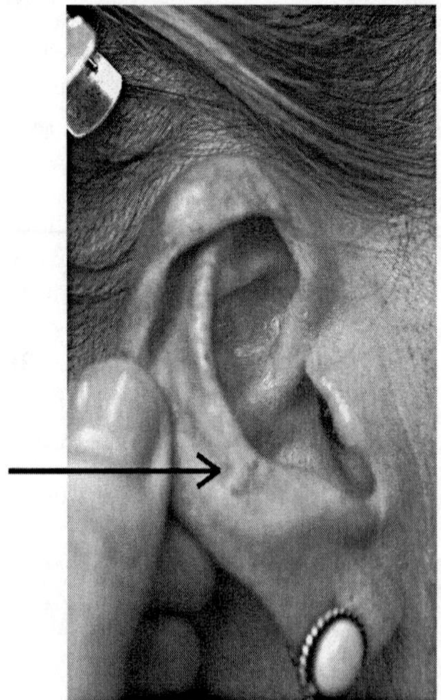

Figure 7.26 Ridge in the Neck area (patient has neck pain).

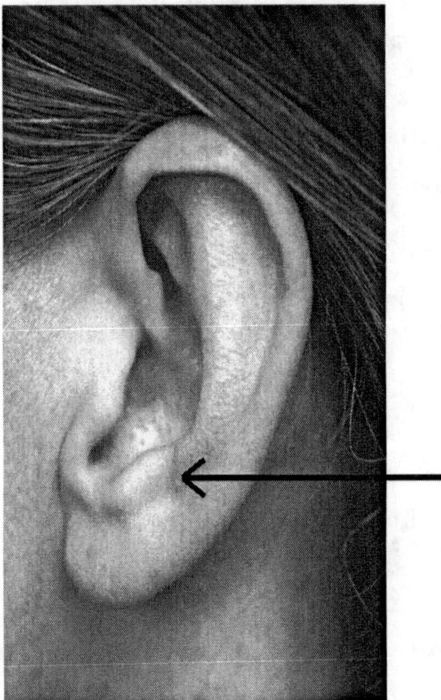

Figure 7.27 Groove at the Cervical point (patient has neck and shoulder tension).

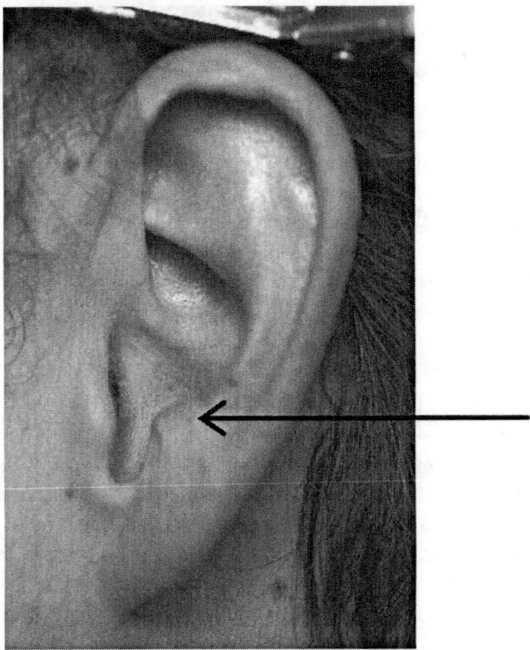

Figure 7.28 The Smart Crest (indicative of high intelligence).

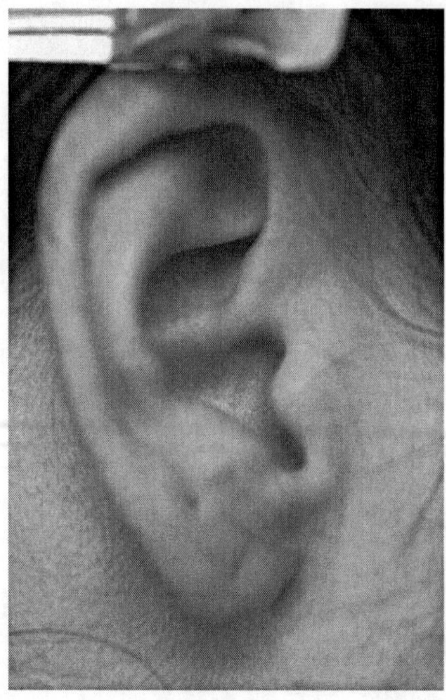

Figure 7.29 Pathological lumpy ear (a good ear to benefit from massage).

References

1. Porkert, M. *The Essentials of Chinese Diagnostics*. Chinese Medicine Publications, Zurich, Switzerland, 1983, p. 166.
2. Romoli, M., Tordini, G., and Giommi, A. Diagonal ear-lobe crease: possible significance as cardiovascular risk factor and its relationship to ear acupuncture. *Acupunc. Electrother. Res.*, 1989, 14(2): 149–154.
3. Kushi, M. *Oriental Diagnosis*. Sunwheel Publications, London, U.K., 1978, pp. 35–36.
4. Porkert, M. *The Essentials of Chinese Diagnostics*. Chinese Medicine Publications, Zurich, Switzerland, 1983, p. 166.

Bibliography

Chen, W.C. Ear lobe crease, high serum cholesterol and human leukocytic antigen risk factors in coronary artery disease. *Chin. Med. J.*, Nov. 1982, 95(11): 839.

Christiansen, J.S. et al. Diagonal ear lobe crease in coronary heart disease. *N. Eng. J. Med.*, 1975, 293: 308.

Frank, S.T. Aural sign of coronary artery disease. *N. Eng. J. Med.*, 1973, 289: 327.

Huang, H. (trans.). *Nanking Army Ear Acupuncture Team*. Rodale Press, Emmaus, PA, 1974.

Kaukola, B. Ear lobe crease and coronary atherosclerosis, *Lancet*, 1979, 2: 1377.

Kushi, M. *Oriental Diagnosis*. Sunwheel Publications, London, U.K., 1978.

Lichstein, E., Chadda, K.D., Naik, D.N., and Gupta, P.K. Diagonal ear-lobe crease; prevalence and implications as a coronary risk factor. *N. Eng. J. Med.*, 1974, 290(11): 615–616.

Mehta, J. and Hamby, R.I. Diagonal ear lobe crease as a coronary risk factor. *N. Eng. J. Med.*, 1974, 29: 260.

Petrakis, N. Earlobe crease in women: evaluation of reproductive factors, alcohol use, and quetelet index and relation to atherosclerotic disease. *Am. J. Med.*, 1995, 99: 356–361.

Porkert, M. *The Essentials of Chinese Diagnostics.* Chinese Medicine Publications, Zurich, Switzerland, 1983.

Rhoads, G.G. et al. The ear lobe crease sign of obesity in middle aged Japanese. *Hawaii Med. J.*, 1977, 36: 74.

Romoli, M., Tordini, G., and Giommi, A. Diagonal ear-lobe crease: possible significance as cardiovascular risk factor and its relationship to ear-acupuncture. *Acupunc. Electrother. Res.*, 1989, 14(2): 149–154.

Sternlieb, J.J. et al. The ear crease in coronary artery disease. *Circulation*, 1974, 50: 152.

Still, J. and Konrad, J. Diagnostic ear acupuncture in the dog; the relationship between active points and internal and skin diseases. *Am. J. Acupunc.*, Jan.–Mar. 1987, 15(1): 53–60.

Still, J. Role of the nervous system in the appearance of ear acupuncture point in the dog: *Acta Veta. Hung.*, 1986, 55(2): 55–64, (in Hungarian).

Taubert, K. Diagnosis using the ear. *Z. Arztl. Fortbild.*, Oct. 12, 1992, 86(19): 945–946, (in German).

Troshin, O.V. Auricular diagnosis of cochleovestibular disorders. *Ross. Med. Z.*, 1992, 1: 27-29, (in German).

chapter eight

Ear prescriptions: construction and formulae for specific conditions

Objective

- To learn the parameters of ear treatment efficacy
- To learn the general rules of ear acupuncture prescriptionology
- To understand ear point prescription formation by studying standardized ear acupuncture prescriptions for common clinical conditions
- To understand the clinical usage of ear acupuncture points by studying specific clinical cases

Part I: constructing ear prescriptions

A fundamental premise of Oriental medical theory is to treat what one sees. By doing so the practitioner has the opportunity to address the whole patient as expressed through his or her unique energetic pattern. Although some practitioners of auricular acupuncture maintain that there is no need for neither diagnosis nor prescription construction, but only adherence to set formulae for specific conditions, this is generally not the Oriental medical viewpoint.

The goal of this chapter is to illustrate to the practitioner how to construct an ear prescription that meets the treatment needs of the patient. While each specific patient will receive a unique formula, the logic of prescription construction needs to be explained. First, however, we need to keep in mind that the ultimate efficacy of a prescription is related to all of the features discussed.

Ear treatment efficacy

Correct diagnosis and treatment plan

Before selecting points or beginning treatment, establish a working diagnosis of the patient's illness in Oriental medical terms. A treatment plan can then be established. For instance, if the patient has a headache at the vertex and you have correctly differentiated this type headache as Liver *Yang* Rising, the treatment plan then is to subdue the Liver *Yang*.

Correct point selection according to the energetics that correspond to the diagnosis and treatment plan

Following the establishment of a diagnosis and its related treatment plan, now select points for their best therapeutic value. The energetics of most of the ear points can be chosen from an understanding of Oriental medical theory. In the case listed above concerning the headache at the vertex, select possible points such as the Ear Apex point (which reduces Liver *Yang)* and the Liver point (to adjust the Liver).

As is true with body acupuncture treatment of illness, the inclusion of ear points that addresses etiological factors assists in a more long-lasting resolution of the problem. Consider the application of this criterion to the Liver *Yang* Rising headache. First, we must determine the etiology of the Liver *Yang* Rising. Is the Liver Yang Rising due to Liver *Yin* Deficiency, Liver Blood Deficiency, Kidney *Yin* Deficiency, or Earth counteracting on Wood? Points are selected according to the specific etiology of the patient's problem. For instance, add the Spleen and Stomach points if the headache is due to Earth counteracting on Wood, the Kidney point if the headache is due to Kidney *Yin* Deficiency, and so forth.

Dr. Chen Gongsun[1] points out that an increase in the therapeutic effect of auricular therapy can be gained if one selects a few but good points. He says:

> Some practitioners favor the use of seeds on 20 to 30 points or more on one ear for each treatment. This form of treatment is likened to "assembling troops to destroy the enemy." It is effective for certain diseases. However, a disadvantage of this form of treatment is that there is no specific focus on a particular disease, and it increases the suffering and apprehension of patients. When so many points are used, we cannot determine whether they have a synergistic or antagonistic effect on each other, nor is it clear which point is the main one. Therefore, I concur with the majority of auricular point practitioners that less than four points should be used in each treatment. In general, I subscribe to the use of points on one side sufficient to treat the disease; in fact, for certain diseases, e.g., gastrospasm, sprains, and pain in the fingers, the stimulation of a single auricular point is enough to obtain a good

> result. The number of points used does not determine the outcome of the treatment. The principle of selecting a few good points guarantees a good result."

Personally I concur with Dr. Gongsun that we should limit the number of points to be treated in the ear. This will come about naturally if we avoid a symptomatic approach and instead correctly differentiate the syndrome and address etiological factors. It is true that there are times when the one well-chosen point is all that is needed, particularly in cases of pain or disorders with musculoskeletal involvement. For the most part, my typical prescription is about seven to eight points.

Accurate point location

After correct point selection, accurate point location must be achieved. You should be able to define where all the points are. This verbal ability will reinforce your adeptness at location. Study the ear maps and point location descriptions found in Chapter 3, and, most importantly, practice to become proficient at point location by using the ear for treatment. The map presented in this book is traditional, time-tested, and easy to learn and to remember and master.

Appropriate ear modality chosen

Many ear modalities are interchangeable, such as seeds, tacks, pellets, and magnets. Others are a matter of personal or cultural preference, such as massage or needles. Still other modalities are highly correlated with a treatment plan, a diagnosis, a clinical disorder, or the "nature" or physiology of the point. For instance, if the point is more of an area, such as the Sacral Vertebrae or the Constipation area, an intradermal can be more effective because an intradermal stimulates the entire area vs. a specific point. In another instance, if Heat or Fire is present, bleeding is the preferred modality to remove the Heat or Fire. Review Chapter 6 and Table 6.1 for the modalities that are correlated with various conditions.

Correct angle of insertion of needles and intradermals if chosen as a modality

The most common angle of insertion into an ear point is perpendicular. Others are needled at an oblique angle. The angle is usually dictated by the anatomical location of the point, so think about physical access when needling the point. For instance, the Brain point, which is located on the posterior aspect of the antitragus, cannot be needled perpendicularly. One needs to needle obliquely behind the antitragus towards the point.

Apart from physical access into the point, *The Nanking Army Acupuncture Book* says that "clinical experience has shown that the angle of insertion into a point may relate to its effectiveness."[2] In the event that the desired results are not being met, you can change the angle of insertion to increase the effectiveness of the point. These angles of insertion have not been standardized by any practitioner because there are so many degrees at which the point could potentially be needled. So, if required, experiment and gain your own clinical experience with that point for each patient.

Da Qi *sensation obtained in the ear, especially of heat*

The degree of ear treatment effectiveness has been correlated with the *Da Qi* sensation obtained in the ear. While there are various signs of *Qi* arrival, clinically the sensation of heat perceived by the patient has been shown to be the most effective variable for successful ear treatment. Try to obtain this through accurate point location, best insertion angle, needle technique, and patient perception and feedback.

Patient's condition and compliance with the modalities

Of course, we must always keep in mind that we are not the healer of an illness. With our expertise, we can certainly help to redirect *Qi* (energy) according to the natural laws of life; however, healing does not always occur, and we must accept that fact. The patient's life force may be beyond our ability to reach with ear modalities. Some diseases will be easy to treat, some impossible, and with others the results might be limited.

Another important factor involved in healing is patient compliance. To enhance compliance, inform your patients of the treatment plan and prognosis, and provide them with written instructions of all directives. However, recognize that some variables are beyond our control as practitioners. The patient may not keep appointments or change certain lifestyle factors. Personal resources (i.e., money, transportation, social support for treatment) are oftentimes limited, as is the ability to follow self-treatment instructions.

Correct construction of the ear prescription

As Joseph Helms states, "Auricular acupuncture can serve as a therapeutic input for disorders on any level of manifestation, and anywhere along the material-to-energetic presentation spectrum."[3] This is a reminder that more than physical maladies can be treated with ear acupuncture. Point selection in both body acupuncture and auricular acupuncture is an art because it is based upon the uniqueness of each patient. Therefore, the practitioner must be able to look at the deeper web of physiological and energetic symptoms and decipher them. Still there are guidelines that enter into the formulation of an ear acupuncture prescription that need to be considered.

How to construct an ear prescription

Start with Shenmen *unless contraindicated*

Unless the patient has bronchitis, bronchial asthma, or congestive heart failure (conditions characterized by excess Phlegm in the chest, which can interfere with respiration), begin the treatment with *Shenmen. Shenmen* quiets the Heart, calms the spirit, and puts the patient into a state of receptivity for treatment. *Shenmen* anchors the spirit before the *Qi* is tonified or dispersed. This is an extremely important treatment principle according to the Three Treasures paradigm, which maintains that of the three treasures — *Qi, Shen,* and *Jing* — the *Shen* (Spirit) must be treated first. *Shenmen* has multiple energetics. It is useful in pain control, in reducing anxiety and restlessness, and in controlling the Blood.

Keep the prescription simple: select primary points for the disorder

The Chinese maintain that each point acts specifically without disturbing the other points; therefore, it is possible to use several points in an ear prescription. However, the Chinese also assert that "it would appear that well-chosen points, even one point, can give more specific results than multistimulation."[4]

Start with one major point to treat the disorder. For instance, if the patient has a respiratory problem:

- *Shenmen* may or may not be indicated. If Phlegm is present, *Shenmen* is prohibited. Otherwise, *Shenmen* could be an excellent point to reduce the anxiety that often accompanies respiratory problems.
- Choose a Lung point as pivotal to the prescription because the Lungs are the anatomical and physiological organ responsible for respiration. Then, round out the balance of the prescription.
- The Kidney point can be added to the prescription to facilitate deep breathing and enhance the ability of the Lungs to descend and disperse the *Qi* so that the Kidney will grasp the *Qi.*
- The Sympathetic point aids in increasing vasodilation (if air pathways are constricted), balances the autonomic nervous system, and reduces any pain associated with the problem, such as tightness in the chest.
- To reinforce the treatment, *Dingchuan* and Stop Wheezing points work well together if there is a pronounced problem with inhalation, otherwise, one or the other can be selected.
- The Diaphragm point is used to open the chest, make the auricle more sensitive to treatment, spread Liver *Qi,* and balance the three *Jiaos*, which are in disharmony.
- Again for reinforcement, the Brain or Brainstem points can further assist in regulating respiration.
- Chest, Inner nose, and/or Trachea can be added to treat localized symptoms and reinforce the treatment based upon the specific locale of the respiratory problem.

As in preparing an herbal formula, consider the interaction between the ear points and how the formula works as a whole to treat the condition. For instance, the Lung point works harmoniously with the Kidney point because of their *Zang-fu* and Five Element interrelationships.

In contrast to synergistic relationships, some points work antagonistically against each other. For instance, I have found that the Antifatigue point (also called the Mouth point) can interfere with the Insomnia point because of their opposite actions. For instance, let us say that a patient has insomnia and, therefore, is tired during the day and may desire more energy. As the practitioner, you chose the Insomnia point to promote sleep and the Mouth point for its antifatigue effects. The most important point to use here is the Insomnia point. Then, when the patient gets enough sleep, he will not be as tired during the day. But if you do use both points, be aware that if you have the person rub the Mouth point at night, the resulting stimulation may keep him awake. Instead, the Insomnia point should be rubbed gently before going to bed, but not too vigorously or it may keep the patient awake.

I prefer to prescribe less ear points and instead treat the root of the patient's particular variety of insomnia. For instance, if the basis of the disorder is insomnia due to Heart *Yin* Deficiency, then choose the Heart point. If the root of the insomnia is due to fullness in the Stomach, then choose the Stomach point. This holds true for treating the etiology of their fatigue as well, which could have numerous origins.

Choose powerful points with multiple functions

Choose points with powerful multiple functions, such as Brain, Sympathetic, Adrenal, Vagus, Diaphragm, Occiput, and Brainstem. I typically add Brain to many formulae because the brain regulates the entire body. The Brain point tends to be tender on palpation because it controls everything. Sympathetic is central to many formulae when the patient is experiencing pain or an imbalance in the autonomic nervous system. Similarly, the Diaphragm Point is an important point for harmonizing the ear acupuncture formula, and connecting all three *Jiaos*. Because these points possess multiple energetics, they are economical to use in the sense of performing several functions.

Add points that treat the root of the disorder and augment the prescription with points that treat symptoms originating from the root

Select points that get at the root of the problem. Do not just think symptomatically. For instance, if a skin problem is due to hypersensitivity to an allergen, add the Liver point to promote the free flowingness of *Qi*. If the skin disorder is due to an autoimmune problem, choose Kidney, which is the foundation of immunity. Add other points based upon signs and symptoms. For instance, if the skin problem is characterized by itchiness, pain, and inflammation, add the Sympathetic point for its ability to treat these characteristics.

Select points based upon the location of the organ, body part, or disease to direct the treatment

Points are selected based upon the location of the organ, body part, or disease that is affected. Use these points as core points or to reinforce a prescription. For example, if there is acne on the skin of the forehead, select the Forehead point. If there is eczema on the cheek, select the Cheek point. Other points would be chosen depending upon the precise location of the problem. If the problem relates to a spinal segment, such as back pain in the lumbar area, Lumbar vertebrae are some of the first points to select.

Do not use points redundantly, but use points to reinforce when needed

An economy of points allows access to the unique energetics of the points and avoids multistimulation. However, there are times when reinforcement is a good and necessary option. For instance, if the person has severe intestinal cramps, you could treat the large intestine through the Large Intestine point, and the Abdomen point can be chosen for reinforcement. But, if you are treating diffuse abdominal pains, the Abdomen point may be sufficient.

Use clinically effective points, which are points with known, proven effectiveness

Clinically effective points, which are points derived from research, have known, proven effectiveness in the treatment of various disorders. They are important points to consider in an ear acupuncture prescription. Such points include the Lumbago point for low back pain; the Lung point for smoking addictions, weight loss, and ulcers; and *Shenmen* for addictions, weight loss, and anxiety. Journal articles are an excellent venue for keeping abreast of the latest research in this specialized field of medicine.

Part II: prescriptions for specific conditions

Obviously, each illness is distinguished by its own signs and symptoms. However, many diseases that are part of a system, such as asthma, bronchitis, cold or allergies, which all affect the respiratory system, share common features. These symptoms include tightness in the chest, difficulty breathing, cough and so forth. As a result, I have created a number of protocols constituting a broad, yet common, treatment plan that can be used by practitioners for a wide assortment of illnesses. Studying these protocols can assist the practitioner in learning, as well as, how to write prescriptions.

Standardized ear treatment for geriatric patients

A seven-point formula — modify this seven-point formula according to the patient's signs and symptoms if necessary. Add points for specific conditions or localized areas of pain, such as knees, low back, or shoulder.

1. ***Shenmen*** — *Shenmen* quiets the Heart, calms the spirit, and puts the patient into a state of receptivity for the treatment. This point can be used to treat restlessness, insomnia, and mental disorders sometimes characteristic of old age. *Shenmen* neutralizes toxins and cures inflammation, such as arthritis, commonly seen in the elderly. Many geriatric diseases have a pain component. *Shenmen* is one of the most clinically effective points for pain because this point pertains to the Heart and, as the *Neijing* (see Chapter 1, History) says, "When the heart is serene, all pain is negligible."
2. **Sympathetic (any of its three locations)** — the Sympathetic point relieves pain, so it is a useful point if an elderly patient has pain, as many do. The Sympathetic point stimulates dilation of blood vessels, therefore improving circulation (the lack of circulation being a leading cause of illness in the elderly). It is also used to treat opthamological diseases that are common in the elderly.
3. **Kidney** — this point tonifies the Root *Qi* of the body (the foundation *Yin* and *Yang*), which declines with aging.

4\. and 5. **Spleen and Stomach** — treating Spleen and Stomach reinforces post-natal *Qi*, which may be weak in the elderly due to age or poor nutrition. Treating these points builds Blood. Since the Spleen dominates the muscles, it is good for treating muscular atrophy and muscle weakness due to lack of exercise and age.

6. **Brain** — the Brain point regulates neurological function and benefits the mind. This point regulates the excitation or inhibition of the cerebral cortex and is a general treatment point for diseases of the nervous, digestive, endocrine, and urogenital systems. It can be used to treat neuropsychiatric disorders, insomnia, and prolapse. All of the aforementioned problems are common in the elderly.
7. **Liver** — the Liver promotes the free flowingness of *Qi* in the body, thereby maintaining the harmonious relationship between the internal organs and external environments. It moves Blood, moves Stagnation, builds Blood and *Yin*, and increases energy. Blood disorders, especially Blood deficiency, Stagnation, and *Yin* deficiency are common patterns of disharmony in the aged.

Modalities and contraindications

The elderly can benefit from auriculotherapy because the auricular treatment, especially with pellets, is gentle and effective. As always, provide written instructions to enhance patient compliance. However, if the patient has a memory problem, he or she might not be able to follow the ear therapy instructions at home. Do not prescribe home therapy if the patient's mental state or living situation interferes with the patient's ability to follow the instructions.

Standardized treatment for the side effects of cancer treatment

Oncology formula

An eight-point formula — use as follows or add or delete points based on signs and symptoms or specific areas of the body affected.

1. ***Shenmen*** — common sequelae to radiation and chemotherapy treatments are the symptoms of anxiety, palpitations, weakness, and restlessness. *Shenmen* is useful for these discomforting feelings because it neutralizes toxins and reduces inflammation, which are also side effects of Western cancer therapy.
2. **Sympathetic** — pain is usually a symptom of cancer treatment therapies, especially radiation. Sympathetic, as we have discussed, is effective in reducing pain.
3. **Lung (Upper and/or Lower)** — as the Master of the *Qi*, the Lung points increase energy, strengthen *Wei Qi* functioning, and improve respiration and oxygenation by sending their energy to the Kidneys. Oncology patients usually report fatigue as their major complaint. The Lung points move the Liver (metal controls wood) and, thus, assist in pain relief. These points relieve depression that is common in patients with serious illness such as cancer. The Lung points aid in treating skin problems due to decreased wound healing capacity and relieve dry and irritated skin. The Lung points are especially helpful in treating skin problems that result from radiation therapy.
4. **Liver** — Liver promotes the free flowingness of *Qi*, maintains the internal patency of *Qi*, and regulates the relationship between the patient's internal and external environments. Liver moves *Qi* and Blood (which may be Stagnant), and balances the emotions. Because cancer is such a devastating illness, the patient's emotions are highly involved in the illness (vs. the emotional component of, say, having a common cold). Liver builds *Yin* and Blood. Radiation patients develop *Yin* deficiency and chemotherapy patients develop *Qi* and Blood deficiency.
5. **Kidney** — the Kidney point tonifies the root *Qi* of the body, the basis of immunity, and builds Blood and *Yin*. It assists in hair regrowth and increases libido. Cancer patients undergoing traditional Western therapies suffer from both hair loss and decreased libido.

6. and 7. **Spleen and Stomach** — Spleen and Stomach reinforce the *Qi* of the *Middle Jiao*; therefore, they are helpful in treating nausea and vomiting, aid digestion, and improve appetite. They reduce Damp/Phlegm, thereby regulating thirst and abdominal distention. The Spleen and Stomach points control the Blood and the Blood vessels and promote the building of Blood, which is necessarily and inevitably damaged along with cancerous cells from Western cancer therapies. These points ground the patient and strengthen the muscles, which are controlled by the Earth element.

8. **Brain (Subcortex)** — the Brain point is used to treat the symptoms of Western cancer treatment, such as fatigue, anxiety, swelling, shock, pain perception, insomnia, and inflammation.

Modalities and contraindications

In my experience of working in an oncology clinic, I found pellets were more effective for cancer patients. Pellets are easy to use, provide continuous therapy at home, and reduce the need for repeated needling, which is contraindicated for weakened patients. Patients must have the pellets removed at the appropriate time in order to minimize the chance of infection. Remember, cancer patients have reduced wound healing capacity.

Standardized pain formula

A seven point formula — for all types of pain. Add other points according to the location of the pain, i.e., shoulder, knee, low back, ovaries, and according to other signs and symptoms.

1. ***Shenmen*** — pain in Oriental medicine is due to stagnation of *Qi*. There are many factors that can lead to this stagnation, such as Heat, Cold, Blood deficiency, and more.[5] The Heart according to *Zang-fu* theory governs the Blood and is responsible for its movement. The *Qi* follows the Blood, thus Stagnation and its clinical manifestation of pain can be treated through the use of *Shenmen*, which is analogous to treating the Heart.
2. **Sympathetic** — the Sympathetic point stimulates the dilation of blood vessels, thereby reducing swelling, congestion, and inflammation, common characteristics of pain.
3. **Diaphragm** — this is a major point for treating *Qi* and Blood Stagnation that lead to pain. The Diaphragm point assists breathing, and this moves the *Qi* of the Lungs and Liver by way of the control cycle. The use of the Diaphragm point is equivalent to opening the *Dai* channel, a channel regulating *Qi* and Blood flow throughout the entire body by way of the three *Jiaos*. Use the Diaphragm point to promote homeostasis and redirect the Blood back to its proper pathway.
4. **Brain** — the Brain point regulates all body systems thereby reducing pain, shock, and inflammation that are characteristics of pain.
5. **Adrenal** — the Adrenal point is used for pain, shock, and inflammation. It regulates hormones that may be involved in the pain manifestation.
6. **Liver** — Liver promotes free flowingness of *Qi*, thereby regulating the Blood. The lack of such patency produces pain.
7. **Relax muscle** — this is a special point within the Liver area that addresses the muscular component of pain by relaxing the muscles.

Modalities and contraindications

Perform an ear needle treatment in the office to activate the flow of *Qi* and Blood and to reduce pain. Tonify or sedate based upon the characteristics of the pain, i.e., whether coming from excess or deficiency. Do an ear pellet treatment in the opposite ear for treatment at home. Retain the take-home treatment for 3 to 5 days, and have the patient press on the pellet 3 to 5 times a day for 3 to 5 seconds. If the patient is needle sensitive, only needle the Sympathetic point or the point that you think might bring the greatest relief, or simply use pellets. If the patient's complaint is due to a disorder that requires surgery, explain to the patient that the ear modality is being used for pain management until surgery, and has not been provided to mask the pain or to replace surgery. If the pain is in the chest or heart and there is a Phlegm component, do not use *Shenmen*.

Standardized immunity treatment

An eight-point formula — this is an effective formula for immune disorders. Add or delete points based upon signs and symptoms if needed.

1. ***Shenmen*** — in the treatment of immunity, *Shenmen* is an important point to balance and settle the patient, as patients with immune disorders are sensitive and delicate.
2. **Sympathetic** — the use of the Sympathetic point in the treatment of immunity is to improve overall functioning and to reduce the pain that accompanies many immune disorders, such as fibromyalgia and lupus erythematosus.
3. **Lung (Upper and/or Lower)** — the Lung points assist in the treatment of immunity by improving respiration (i.e., oxygenation to the body), and help in the emotional components of immune disorders by moving the *Qi* and, thereby, reducing depression. Patients with immune disorders have systemic *Qi* deficiencies. The Lungs, as the Master of the *Qi*, control the *Qi* of the entire body.
4. **Liver** — the Liver point builds *Yin* and Blood. Patients with weak immunity have Blood and *Yin* deficiencies.
5. **Kidney** — the Kidney point is used to tonify the Root *Qi*, the basis of immunity.

6\. and 7. **Spleen and Stomach** — the Spleen and Stomach points stimulate their respective organs to produce *Qi*, Blood, and *Yin*, which are deficient in immune patients.

8. **Brain (Subcortex)** — the Brain point enhances the functioning of the entire body, which is needed in immune problems.

Note: The four previous formulae all have *Shenmen*, Sympathetic, Brain, and Liver. Three of the formulae used Spleen/Stomach. This demonstrates the multiple energetics of points and how they can be used for different conditions.

The next group of formulae treats other common illnesses. Energetics, except where different, will not be noted here. Use this section to test your understanding of point energetics.

Standardized respiratory formula

1. ***Shenmen*** **(as long as no Phlegm)**
2. **Upper and/or Lower Lung**
3. **Kidney**
4. **Diaphragm**

5\. and 6. **Brain and/or Brainstem**

7. ***Dingchuan***
8. **Affected areas (i.e., nose, chest, etc.)**

Fibrocystic breast disease

1. ***Shenmen***
2. **Sympathetic**
3. **Liver**

4\. and 5. **Spleen/Stomach**

6. **Kidney**
7. **Mammary**
8. **Diaphragm**

Acid reflux disease

1. ***Shenmen***
2. **Sympathetic**

3\. and 4. **Spleen/Stomach**

5. **Liver**
6. **Cardiac Sphincter**
7. **Esophagus**
8. **Lung**
9. **Diaphragm**
10. **Throat**

Peripheral neuropathy

1. ***Shenmen***
2. **Sympathetic**
3. **Liver**
4. **Brain**
5. **Affected areas (i.e., fingers, toes, etc.)**
6. **Affected spinal segment**

Stop smoking

1. ***Shenmen***
2. **Liver**

3. and 4. **Lungs (Upper and Lower)**

5. **Kidney**
6. **Mouth**
7. **Stomach**

Prescriptions from China

Prevention of disease: the Nanking Army ear acupuncture prescription

A simple and efficacious auricular acupuncture prescription for the prevention of disease was developed in China in the 1960s. Utilized by the Nanking Army and barefoot doctors during the Cultural Revolution, this formula was designed to strengthen the army's resistance to disease, especially pernicious pathogens, such as malaria, epidemic influenza, and mumps. The Nanking Army protocol is now considered a "prevention of disease" treatment.

In this study, the first company (who received this treatment every 10 days over a course of 12 treatments) had an annual malaria rate of 1.2% in contrast to the second company who had an annual rate as high as 8.5%. Of the group who received ear acupuncture, 80% showed an increase in appetite, improvement in sleep, and strengthened resistance. Those who were treated rarely caught a cold or suffered influenza.[6]

Points	Functions
Suprarenal (also known as Adrenal)	Regulates the hormones of the suprarenal gland, thereby treating infection, inflammation, and shock Regulates blood pressure Reduces fever and heat
Internal Secretion (also known as Triple Warmer)	Regulates internal secretions. Stimulates body fluids (*Jinye*) that contain humoral messages that are part of the immune response Harmonizes the three *Jiaos* Promotes digestion and absorption
Dermis (also known as Lung)	Oxygenates the blood; promotes circulation Regulates body temperature Strengthens the *Qi* (the Lungs are the Master of the *Qi*) and reinforces the *Qi* of the Lungs to protect against exogenous invasion and to enhance systemic *Qi*
Spleen	Controls the Blood, circulates the Blood Strengthens digestion Nourishes the muscles Strengthens the *Qi*

Points	Functions
Liver	For iron deficient anemia Dispels Evil Winds by moving the *Qi* Facilitates the digestive process to support postnatal *Qi* production Moves Liver excess

The strength of this formula lies in its ability to prevent disease. Together these points strengthen the antipathogenic factor (the true *Qi* of the body). However, the prescription can also be used with good results when a patient has an illness such as the flu or the common cold.

The Nanking Army formula is ideal for those who are weak, immunodeficient, dislike needles, or who are very young or elderly. The prescription may be used alone or as a supplement to other treatments. Needles can be used daily or Magrain gold pellets applied to the points every 3 to 5 days for as long as necessary. You should find this formula helpful in your practice.

Other formulas from China

On my first study tour to China in 1988, I saw ear acupuncture used as a primary and independent modality on a large-scale basis. Patients, who expressed their dislike of needles (particularly women, teenagers, and the elderly), preferred this modality of treatment. A list of prescriptions that was used repetitively for the most common clinical conditions is provided below. The reader is encouraged to consult these formulae and try to infer why each point was selected.

Gallstones

Shenmen
Liver
Spleen
Stomach
Brain
Hypertension groove
Sympathetic
Vagus

Myopia

Shenmen
Occiput
Liver
Spleen
Stomach
Heart

Kidney
Lung
Eye
Eye 1 and 2

Stop smoking (three different formulae)

(A)
Shenmen
Upper and Lower Lung
Brain
Adrenal

(B)
Shenmen
Mouth
Spleen
Stomach
Adrenal
Upper or Lower Lung

(C)
Endocrine
Adrenal
Hunger
Infection
Outer Ear (helix)
Adrenal
Occiput
Kidney

Breast disorders/fibrocystic breasts or breast distention

Mammary
Stomach
Endocrine

Insomnia

Shenmen
Heart
Kidney
Brain

Hiccup

Diaphragm

Gastralgia

Shenmen
Stomach
Duodenum
Abdomen

Leukorrhea

Endocrine
Kidney
Ovary

Headache

Shenmen
Brain

Weight loss (three different formulae)

(A)
Shenmen
Stomach
Lower Lung
Hunger

(B)
Shenmen
Endocrine

(C)
Stomach
Brain
Hunger
Thirst

Clinical applications

- ***Dingchuan* and Stop Wheezing** — the patient (student) was a 56-year-old female who had severe asthma most of her adult life. She needed an inhaler on a regular basis to help her breathe. One day in class as I was teaching the students about auricular medicine, she experienced an attack. As she reached for her inhaler, I suggested that she let me needle the point *Dingchuan* in her ear. As soon as I did, she immediately was able to breathe easier. To consolidate the treatment, I also needled the Stop Wheezing point. The student reported that she no longer requires her inhaler when she treats herself, even with pellets, on these points.

- **Oncology Formula for the Side Effects of Chemotherapy** — one year when I was supervising a student clinic at an oncology treatment center, we saw a patient who was very tired. She told us that she had confessed to her doctor that she "felt like a slug" and her doctor told her to get used to that feeling because that is how she would feel for the rest of her life. Because Oriental medicine treats the whole person and has known success in enhancing our feelings of well being, I didn't believe that was the way she had to feel now or for the rest of her life. I administered the Standardized Oncology Formula that I had devised as a core treatment for patients who were undergoing chemotherapy and radiation. Gold magrain pellets were placed on the points and retained for about a week. The next week the patient was ecstatic. Her face and voice were animated and her spirit was exuberant. She told us that she no longer felt like a slug, but rather felt like herself and she could not wait to tell her oncologist that she felt her quality of life could return with the help of ear acupuncture. My students and I were humbled that the simple gesture of applying gold pellets to her ear was so beneficial.
- **The Lumbar-Sacral Area** — in the course of treating a patient for a certain complaint, she also reported that her lower back, specifically in the lumbar-sacral region, was always painful. She had sought acupuncture from a renowned practitioner for this problem, but the treatment did not help. When I inspected her ear, I could see broken blood vessels in that portion of the Vertebral points indicating poor circulation in that area. I inserted an intradermal needle in an upward direction through the Lumbar area towards the Sacral vertebrae. Immediately she said her back felt perfect and years later she reports that the problem has never reoccurred.
- **The Prostate Point** — the patient was a middle-aged man who had periodic inflammation of his prostate gland. When this occurred, his symptoms consisted of burning pain in the penis, referred pain in the perineum, incontinence, painful sex with an inability to ejaculate, painful urination, difficulty initiating the stream, urinary urgency and frequency, and night urination. When this occurred, I would treat him on an emergency basis simply by needling the Prostate point in the ear. Within 10 seconds of inserting the needle, he would become peaceful, very relaxed, and even sleepy and relieved of the pain. I would leave the needle in place for about 20 minutes. When he left the office, he no longer had the pain that accompanied his prostatitis.

- **The Lung Point for Skin Disorders** — the patient developed a severe case of dermatitis by working in a very hot and greasy restaurant kitchen as a cook. The skin problem began as a large rash on the medial aspect of the patient's arms, specifically originating at the cubital crease close to Lung 5 (*Chize*), Heart 3 (*Shaohai*), and Pericardium 3 (*Quze*), and spread outward. The skin rash was red, raised, and unbearably itchy, and became worse when at work. Initially the patient consulted a dermatologist who prescribed a cortisone cream for external application. It helped momentarily. The patient could not stop scratching the area and this contributed to making it even itchier and more inflamed. At that point the patient decided to see an acupuncturist. The acupuncturist put together a small ear acupuncture prescription consisting of the Lung point, which controls the skin; *Shenmen* to quiet the Heart and also to treat pain, skin problems, and inflammation; and Sympathetic for the inflammation and pain. Within seconds of application of the needles, the skin itching diminished. The patient left the office with the needles left in place in her ear. They fell out about an hour later. The results of this treatment lasted 5 days. At that point, the patient had another ear acupuncture treatment with the same points and the skin problem was resolved in less than 2 weeks.
- ***Shenmen* for Shock** — following a car accident, a patient arrived at my office. He clearly was not himself. His pupils were dilated, and his eyes were glassy. He spoke in run-on sentences and was clearly disturbed by the accident. He felt he experienced some whiplash, as musculoskeletal pain began to set in. In prioritizing the treatment, I felt he was in shock and needed to be grounded. I inserted a needle into ear *Shenmen* and balanced the treatment with body point Kidney 6 *(Zhaohai)*. As soon as *Shenmen* was needled, he settled down and became quiet and peaceful. Kidney 6 likewise served to bring his energy down and out of his head, to anchor his spirit, and to quell the trauma that he was experiencing. When he left the office, he was back to himself and did not display the symptoms of shock.

References

1. Gongsun, C. Understanding the increase in therapeutic effect in auricular acupuncture. *Int. J. Clin. Acupunc.*, 2001, 12(1): 51–52.
2. Huang, H. *Ear Acupuncture*. Rodale Press, Emmaus, PA, 1974, pp. 13–14, 722.
3. Helms, J. *Acupuncture Energetics: A Clinical Approach for Physicians.* Medical Acupuncture Publishers, Berkeley, CA, 1995, p. 152.
4. *Practical Ear Needling, 3rd ed.* Medicine and Health Publishing Co. Hong Kong, Sept. 1982, p. 110.
5. Gardner–Abbate, S. The differential diagnosis of pain in classical Chinese medicine: unique treatment approaches and acupoint energetics. *Am. J. Acupunc.*, 1996, 24(4): 269–284.
6. Nanking Army Ear Acupuncture Team. Huang, H. (trans.). *Ear Acupuncutre.* Rodale Press, Emmaus, PA, 1974, pp. 13–14.

Bibliography

Chen, G.S., Xing, J.Q., Yu, M., Hu, Z., Zhong, Y.M., Xu, R.Z., Xu, D., and Zhu, B. The specificity of auricular points – tumor idiosyncrasy regions reflecting cancer diagnosis. *Int. J. Clin. Acupunc.*, 2001, 12(2): 115–122.

Gardner–Abbate, S. The differential diagnosis of pain in classical Chinese medicine: unique treatment approaches and acupoint energetics. *Am. J. Acupunc.*, 1996, 24(4): 269–284.

Gongsun, C. Understanding the increase in therapeutic effect in auricular acupuncture. *Int. J. Clin. Acupunc.*, 2001, 12(1): 51–52.

Helms, J. *Acupuncture Energetics: A Clinical Approach for Physicians.* Medical Acupuncture Publishers, Berkeley, CA, 1995.

Nanking Army Ear Acupuncture Team. Huang, H. (trans.). *Ear Acupuncture.* Rodale Press, Emmaus, PA, 1974.

Practical Ear Needling, 3rd ed., Medicine and Health Publishing Co., Hong Kong, Sept. 1982.

White, A.R., Rampes, H., and Ernst, E. Acupuncture for smoking cessation. *Cochrane Database Sys. Rev.*, 2000, 2.

chapter nine

Clinical research and effective points

Objective

- To review select clinically effective points in the literature search over the past 30 years to appreciate the points' effectiveness when combined with particular auricular modalities

Introduction

Research in the field of auriculotherapy substantiates the effectiveness of ear acupuncture and can inspire the practitioner to use ear acupuncture in many cases, either as the primary mode to treatment or, at least, as a supplementary option. Many studies[1] demonstrate ear acupuncture's effect on conditions such as:

- Pain control
- Respiratory problems
- Circulatory disorders
- Digestive problems
- Urological diseases
- Gynecological and obstetrical illnesses
- Pediatric diseases
- Otolaryngolic illnesses
- Ophthalmologic disorders
- Dermatologic disorders
- Diseases of the nervous system
- Acute abdominal diseases
- Reduction in body weight
- Abstinence in smoking and drinking

Continued research is being done in many areas of the field and the practitioner is encouraged to keep abreast of studies, particularly as presented by journals in the profession as well as to document his or her own cases studies.

In this chapter, the conclusions of several studies done in the field of auricular acupuncture are highlighted. Such research includes the use of the specific effective auricular points and the modalities used in these treatments. The material is organized according to specialties in auricular acupuncture that the practitioner can find useful in his clinical practice. Studies that are redundant are not summarized, only their more differentiating and salient aspects. For more detail as well as an appreciation of the diverse clinical success in many more areas of treatment and the selection of diverse treatment modalities, the reader should consult the original material referenced in the extensive bibliography that is found at the end of each chapter (particularly this one) that spans more than a 30-year period and close to 800 entries.

Weight reduction

The preponderance of early literature on ear acupuncture centered on the topics of weight reduction, drug withdrawal, and pain control. As a result, this has been the common impression that the public and medical doctors have on the applicability of ear acupuncture, although as we have seen, its usefulness is almost unlimited. The overall conclusion from such studies unequivocally supports the use of auricular acupuncture to treat these difficult-to-treat disorders. There are certainly limitations to its use, however. These behavioral problems have complex and intricate social, cultural, physical, and emotional components. The value of auricular acupuncture is clearly evident, however, and it can be used as a valuable part of weight reduction, drug withdrawal, or pain control plans.

The Stomach point is obviously a point to incorporate into the treatment of obesity and weight loss. Apostolos Apostolopoulos[2] explains, "The organ points are found within the vagal zone, which has a parasympathetic innervation. The regional action of the Stomach point is related to the vagus nerve. As such, the Stomach point serves to reduce of motility of the stomach in particular and of the digestive tract in general. On the other hand, it also has the effect of reducing the secretion of gastric acid, which is under the control of the sympathetic nervous system. The clinical effects of these actions diminish the sense of hunger."

Other studies corroborate this concept. "Not only does acupuncture stimulate the auricular branch of the vagus nerve, but it also raises serotonin levels, both of which have been shown to increase tone in the smooth muscle of the stomach, thus suppressing appetite. In one particular study, 95% of overweight subjects noticed suppression of appetite when electric stimulation was applied to the *Shenmen* and Stomach points. No participants in the control group noticed such a change. The study concluded that frequent stimulation of specific auricular points is an effective method of appetite suppression, which leads to weight loss."[3]

In an earlier study by Alkaysi et al.[4] on pathological obesity (defined as weight 20% greater than one's ideal body weight), "Electroacupuncture was applied to the following points: Anus, Ear Apex, Adrenal, Forehead, Temple, Tooth. The explanation for the use of these points was not provided in the study. Good results were obtained and the authors concluded that auricular acupuncture stimulation is a suitable method of treating pathological obesity."

Further studies in obesity showed that "points relating to weight loss cause a reduction in insulin at the time of an empty stomach."[5] Weight loss studies also maintain a tenet that makes sense because of the multiple functions of the ear points and demonstrates that auricular treatment is not only symptomatic. B. Xu[6] found, "Not only can weight be lost, but improvement in body function can be obtained."

The conclusion from many weight loss protocols is that Stomach and *Shenmen* are the two primary points involved in weight loss. The Stomach point directly affects Stomach function and controls physiological scenarios that suppress hunger, reduce appetite, and improve overall Stomach organ function. *Shenmen* reduces the anxiety, nervousness, and restlessness associated with weight loss.

Drug withdrawal

In the voluminous studies that have been done on smoking and drug addictions, the preponderance of them point to the use of two core points, *Shenmen* and Lung, as necessary to treatment. *Shenmen* reduces withdrawal symptoms, such as restlessness, nervousness, anxiety, and cravings. It has a stabilizing effect. The major action of the Lung point is to decrease lethargy, which can develop when the use of stimulants is denied. Because the Lung is the master of the *Qi,* the energy of the body is increased through its use. Thus, the body's own natural ability to regulate proper energy is stimulated.

Researchers H.L. Wen and A.Y.C. Chung first developed a clinical protocol for treating drug withdrawal by using electrical stimulation of the ear. Later, a study using two needles on each ear found "Lung to regulate energy, and Liver to address alcoholism, plus other points based on withdrawal symptoms, to be central to drug detoxification."[7]

The treatment of drug addiction is complex due to the cultural, social, and physiological variables associated with addiction. Auricular medicine is a simple, easy, relatively convenient, and cost-effective treatment to assist in the difficult withdrawal process. W. M. Niu et al.[8] showed that "the short-term curative effect in groups receiving electroacupuncture combined with ear pressing therapy was found to be equivalent to groups treated by methadone maintenance. However, the reoccurrence rate in patients treated with ear acupuncture is significantly lower." An Avants et al.[9] study between cocaine dependent patients and methadone-maintained patients showed that "cocaine use decreased significantly for patients receiving body acupuncture or ear acupuncture compared with the methadone maintenance group."

The National Acupuncture Detoxification Association (NADA) has popularized the use of ear acupuncture in drug detoxification in the U.S. and abroad. The NADA five-point protocol utilizes *Shenmen*, Sympathetic, Kidney, Liver, and Lung to treat narcotic, alcohol, and nicotine addiction. The energetics of those points in the detoxification protocol should be apparent now that the energetics of the points have been discussed throughout this book. Those clinicians trained as specialists in the NADA protocol have completed a great deal of successful work and helped many thousands of patients suffering from the enslavement of various addictions. Addiction withdrawal is not my area of ear expertise, so it is best to directly consult the literature and studies done with this procedure if the reader has interest in this important area of treatment.

Smoking is also an addictive behavior. Tiziano Marovino[10] reports, "After using laser auriculotherapy for nicotine detoxification, 48% of the subjects still were not smoking 3 months later. However, they were intrinsically motivated individuals who did not have high stress levels. The laser was employed to minimize the withdrawal symptoms — not to cure the entire biopsychosocial constellation of variables that are inherent in any type of addiction."

X.S. Liu's[11] study, using semen vaccaria, showed that "ear treatment affects the sense of taste. Cigarette smoke tastes bitter and undesirable to smokers once they begin ear treatment, thus reinforcing the undesirability of the habit."

Pain control and burn trauma

Relieving the complex process of pain that is part of the human condition has been a focus in medicine, and ear acupuncture is no exception. In almost all types of pain that do not require surgical intervention, Oriental medicine and ear acupuncture have been highly successful in the remediation of pain. Auricular acupuncture can be selected as a modality of choice to assist in pain control, pain reduction, and even remediation, if the causative factors are acknowledged. If points are selected carefully according to the diagnosis and if ear point location and needle technique are correct, pain may be alleviated in a matter of seconds to hours. In my experience, I have found that the more acute the pain, the faster it can be relieved vs. chronic pain, which takes longer due to lingering etiological factors.

Hua Sun[12] writes, "Comparisons of randomized patients assigned to receive body acupuncture vs. auricular acupuncture had an effective rate for the auricular acupuncture group that surpasses the body acupuncture group and that the difference was statistically significant."

H. Wu et al.[13] say that "in treating postoperative pain due to incisions, auricular medicine was successful over analgesics, which have several side effects. The operations included gall bladder removal, appendectomy, radical open colon and rectal operations, hernia repair, thyroidectomy, removal of mammary tumor, and subgastrectomy. The reason advanced for this is that auricular pressing dredges the channels, thus the stasis can be removed and the pain diminished."

Beatrice Umeh[14] points out, "In patients suffering from acute torticollis, a Nigerian study showed significant relief for patients within 24 hours by way of ear tacks. The researcher also concluded that tropical weather did not increase the chances of ear infection, although getting the ear wet did."

In the management of pain and inflammation that are a sequel to burn trauma, E. Jichova and associates[15] found "*Shenmen* and the thalamic projection points were effective in pain mitigation. They supplemented the treatment with body points LU 7 (*Lieque*), LI 4 (*Hegu*), and ST 36 (*Zusanli*)." This is a useful modality to consider because of the debilitating nature of burn pain and the limited modalities that acupuncturists have at their disposal to treat those patients.

Sports medicine and musculoskeletal disorders

As mentioned in Chapter 1, musculoskeletal disorders benefit from treatment with auricular acupuncture. From the area of sports medicine have come several studies that choose the ear for treatment. J. G. Lin and associates[16] found that "using ear point pressing therapy with semen vaccaria, auriculotherapy was effective for increasing oxygen levels and lowering the lactic acid buildup that follows exercise. Some points that were effective include the Liver point, Lung point, Subcortex, Endocrine, and Triple Warmer. The Liver point assists the regulation of blood volume and Liver function, such as the nutrients used during muscular activity. The Liver point simulates the Liver to remove lactic acid via metabolism or conversion. The Lung point aids nervous, digestive, and cardiovascular systems, and also modulates the function of the cerebral cortex and increases oxygen uptake. The Subcortex point affects the cerebral cortex that governs the entire body, the Endocrine point regulates the endocrine system, and the Triple Warmer point controls all the visceral organs."

In analyzing the functions of these points, it is seen that they pertain to the organs integral to physiological functioning during exercise and recovery. The authors[16] also concluded, "In addition to these findings, overall, volunteers felt more comfortable during exercise. This has possible implications for longer and more intensive training, if desired. This study contains an excellent and understandable exposition on exercise physiology using both Western and Oriental paradigms."

Polio

In the U.S. alone there are approximately 75,000 post-polio patients. Most physicians today have not seen acute poliomyelitis in their practices because polio was an epidemic in the 1950s and polio's presence in the modern world is almost nonexistent. Currently a new variant, called post-polio syndrome (PPS) is present in about 25% of the polio population.

Post-polio syndrome is a constellation of symptoms that develop about 20 to 25 years after acute onset of polio in survivors. It is characterized by unaccustomed fatigue, joint and muscle pain, muscle weakness, loss of muscle use, respiratory problems, depression, and other criteria.

In a PPS ear study, points employed were *Shenmen*, Upper Cervical Vertebrae, Occiput (Atlas), Brain, Lumbar Vertebrae, Sympathetic Ganglion, Vagus Nerve, Diaphragm (point O), Ipsilateral (same side) Lung, Heart, plus additional local points. Using bilateral electrical stimulation, good to excellent results were obtained, with 66.7% of participants reporting a return to preexisting levels of health. According to F. Doubler,[17] this study appears to be the first effective, permanent, relatively simple, and inexpensive form of therapy for the treatment of post-polio syndrome.

Mental health

Depressive states, hallucinations, anxiety, psychosomatic disorders, and mental retardation

In an interesting study by G. B. H. Lewis,[18] on the use of oral diazepam, ear acupuncture and a relaxation tape were compared as methods of controlling preoperative anxiety. Both of the nondrugless options were easy to use and suggest advantages over drugs when rapid recovery is desired. The point used was Wexu's Relaxing Zone — also known as the Chinese Nervousness (anxiety) point, Nogier's Aggressivity point, or Oleson's Worry Master Controller point. It is located along the margins of the medial border of the lobe in the infratragal area. This same point was also found to be more effective than *Shenmen* in S. M. Wang and Z. N. Kain's[19] study in significantly reducing anxiety in a normal volunteer population (i.e., did not have preoperative anxiety). The study concluded that the use of the Anxiety point helped in the regulation of anxiety prior to surgery.

"In 120 people suffering hallucinations and treated with auricular acupuncture, an 80% success rate was achieved in treating schizophrenia, reactive psychosis, senile psychosis, and climacteric disorder using the Anxiety point (discussed above), Subcortex, and External Auricle in the first treatment, and *Shenmen*, *Yangwei*, and Internal Ear in the second treatment."[20]

In another study by M. Romoli and A. Giommi,[21] "Patients with possible psychosomatic disorders of the cardiovascular, respiratory, and digestive systems were treated with ear acupuncture. It was found that the point most sensitized to stress was the Triple Warmer or *Sanjiao* point." This study emphasizes the importance of *Sanjiao* as a treatment point for clinical usage including psychosomatic disorders.

According to evaluation by standard IQ tests, L. Tian[22] claims that "128 children with mental retardation had an improvement in intelligence quotient (IQ) and social adaptation behavior (SAB) when treated with acupuncture, auriculo-pellet pressure, and herbal plasters on acupoints."

Gastric disorders, cholelithiasis

Biliary colic is a common and painful condition. Its treatment frequently requires intramuscular injections of conventional analgesics, which cause numerous side effects. In a study by Y. Zhang and associates[23] done on rabbits, it was found that "marked contraction of the gall bladder occurs after only 1 minute of stimulation of the Gall Bladder point, thus proving that the Gall Bladder point corresponds to the gall bladder in rabbits. The contraction lasted for 30 to 40 minutes."

In another study[24] on the clinical effectiveness of ear acupuncture needles for biliary colic, a success rate of 93.33% was obtained. The only point used in this study was *Erzhong* or the Diaphragm Point (also known as Point Zero by Nogier and the Master Point by Oleson). Pain was relieved in 2 to 5 minutes by twirling the needle for 15 seconds every 3 to 5 minutes. Hiccups, jaundice, infantile enuresis, dermatitis, diseases of the digestive tract, diaphragmatic spasm, and kidney and gastrointestinal colic also were found to be relieved by this point.

Z. Y. Li and colleagues'[25] study found ear seed therapy to be 86.5% successful in eliminating gallstones. A 1989 study[26] had a 70% success rate in expelling gallstones from the Liver and Gallbladder along with the patient eating a lard-fried egg every day to activate the Gallbladder. The ear points used were Heart, Brain, Liver, Gallbladder, Kidney, *Shenmen,* and Spleen. with semen vaccaria applied to the points. Motor function of the Gallbladder was initiated within 30 to 45 minutes.

Lung is one of the most clinically effective points for gastric ulcer because the Lungs, by dominating the mucous membranes, heal the lining of the Stomach.

Gynecological problems

Climacteric disorder and dysmenorrhea

M. L. Wang[27] observed that "for the treatment of symptoms of climacteric syndrome, marked-to-good improvement was obtained in 37 out of 42 cases when the type of disorder was properly differentiated. The primary points used were Kidney, Internal Genitalia, Subcortex, and Endocrine. For Kidney *Yin* Deficiency with Liver *Yang* Rising, Lung, Liver, and Spleen were added. For Kidney *Yin* Deficiency with disharmony of the Heart and Kidney, Liver, Heart, and *Shenmen* were used. For Kidney *Yin* and *Yang* deficiency with Spleen weakness, the Spleen and Small Intestine points were included. If hypertension presented, the Hypertension groove and Liver points were added. Pellets were retained in the ear for 3 days. Six sessions constituted a course of treatment and three courses were the average treatment time."

D. Lewers et al.[28] study on the treatment of primary dysmenorrhea resulted in an average pain relief of at least 50% immediately posttreatment using TENS electrostimulation. The study also suggested that auriculotherapy via acupressure may relieve the same pain.

Rheumatoid arthritis

Using ear treatment, R. S. Shapiro and associates[29] found that "the thymus point proved effective in patients with rheumatoid arthritis when using laser therapy. Patients obtained rapid pain relief and improvement in mobility. This suggests that drug reduction and improvement in the quality of life may be achievable in patients suffering from rheumatoid arthritis."

A.B. Zhu and colleagues[30] study performed on experimental rats with acute arthritis showed electrical acupuncture had the therapeutic effect of promoting blood circulation, reducing extravasated blood, antiphlogistic, and detumescence on the area of pathological changes in the rats.

Ear, nose, and throat

Infantile trachitis, esophageal motility, and hiccups

Auricular acupuncture also was a useful therapeutic procedure, Hep et al. reports, in treating impaired motility of the esophagus, a common finding in patients with functional blocks of the cervical spine.[31]

F.L. Li and colleagues'[32] write, "Intractable postsurgical hiccups that can continue for weeks following thoracic and abdominal surgery was effectively treated (95.2%) using ear needles that were retained for 20 to 40 minutes over the course of three treatments. The points treated were *Erzhong* (Diaphragm), *Shenmen*, and Sympathetic as the primary points, and Stomach, Liver, Kidney, Lung, *Yuanzhong*, Thorax, and Abdomen as secondary points."

Coronary artery disease

Angina pectoris, arteriosclerosis, blood pressure, hypertension, and diabetic angiopathy

X. Q. Zhou and J. X. Liu[33] help illustrate the role of auricular acupuncture in the area of cardiology. They demonstrated that ear *Shenmen* and the Heart point played a significant role with just one treatment by reducing the frequency and duration of the symptoms of angina pectoris.

C. Feng et al.[34] point out that "transcranium doppler ultrasound examination revealed increased blood flow rates in the brain with significant differences before and after treatment when ear *Shenmen* was treated with electromagnetic therapy."

Auricular acupoints also can treat hypertension. R. X. Zhou, Y. H. Zhang, and associates[35] illustrated that "a transient antihypertensive effect with semen vaccaria could be achieved for up to 1 month by using 5 to 6 of the following ear points replaced twice a week over a 3 month period: *Shenmen*, Sympathetic, Liver, Heart, Spleen, Kidney, *Erjian* (Ear apex), Lung, Helix 6, Subcortex, and the Hypertension groove. The most effective time to press was found to be before noon. The treatment worked better for females and Type A — *Taiyang*- or Fire-type patients."

H. Q. Huang and S. Z. Liang[36] found "blood pressure was lowered with needling the Heart point. The short-term hypotensive rate was 100% and the forward effective rate was 63.3%." P. I. Gaponiuk and M. V. Leonova[37] discovered that "certain patients with hypertension were able to discontinue drugs and other patients were able to reduce their drug intake."

In the area of diabetes M. N. Solun and A. L. Liaifer[38] report, "In patients with insulin-dependent diabetes mellitus with functional stage of lower limb diabetic angiopathy, body and auricular points were successful. These points enhanced blood outflow and regulation of the lower limb, vascular peripheral resistance, and improved elastotonic properties of arteries of average caliber."

Urinary calculus

Retention

L. Chen[39] used the following points to relieve the symptoms of bladder stones as well as expulsion of the stones: Kidney, Endocrine, Urinary Bladder, and Sympathetic as the main ear points, and Spleen, Triple Warmer, Urethra, Brain, and Ureters as auxiliary points, using the semen vaccaria method.

Q. Wang and Y. Y. Zhao[40] found that "urinary retention due to postoperative anal pain was successfully relieved by needling in the ear. *Shenmen*, Sympathetic, and the center of the triangular fossa were used. The needles were rotated for 1 minute and then rotated until micturition began. The time frame within which micturition began ranged from 5 to 30 minutes after treatment started."

Skin and immunity

Lupus erythematosus

Lupus erthymtosus is a disorder of the skin due to weak immunity. Y. S. Chen and X. I. Hu[41] found that needles applied to points according to signs and symptoms showed good result in the treatment of discoid lupus erythematosus.

Myopia

Myopia is viewed in Oriental medicine as due to congenital insufficiency or bad eye habits. In young adults, H. F. Cheng[42] shows "Myopia was well treated using semen vaccaria on Eye 1, Eye 2, Eye, Occiput, Liver, and Kidney. Three courses of treatment produced a 93% success rate." An H. Liu et al.[43] study reports a 44.3% improvement of adolescents' myopia and a 98.5% increase in visual acuity using semen impatientis. Treatment was administered once a week with four treatments constituting a course of treatment, and one to four courses administered."

A study by C. Yang and colleagues[44] combined ear-pressing therapy with injections of placenta to treat myopia. The placenta injection was used to enhance the semen vaccaria's known efficacy. Placenta has been shown to have good effect in the treatment of strain, constitutional feebleness, and chronic ocular disease. Placenta invigorates *Qi*, nourishes Blood, replenishes body Essence, and, as a tonic, corrects congenital insufficiency and deficiency of *Qi* and Blood.

References

1. Chen, G. Advances in researches in auriculo-acupoints. *J. Trad. Chin. Med.*, 1991, 11(3): 216–233.
2. Apostolopoulos, A. Treatment of obesity and weight loss by auricular acupuncture in 800 cases. *The Medical Acupuncture Web Page*. Announced at ICMART, 1996, VII World Congress, Copenhagen, p. 49.
3. Richards, D. and Marley, J. Stimulation of auricular points in weight loss. *Aust. Fam. Phys.*, Jul. 1998, 27 (Suppl.) 2: 73–77.
4. Alkaysi, G., Leindler, L., Bajusz, H., and Szarvas, F. The treatment of pathological obesity by a new auricular method: a five year clinical experience. *Am. J. Acupunc.*, 1991, 19 (4): 323–328.
5. Mukaino, Y. Acupuncture therapy for obesity using ear needle treatment: analysis of effectiveness and mechanisms of action. *J. Japn. Soc. Acupunc.*, 1981, 31(1): 67–74, (in Japanese).
6. Xu, B. Clinical observation of the weight reducing effect of ear acupuncture in 350 cases of obesity. *J. Trad. Chin. Med.*, 1985, 5(2): 87–88.
7. Wen, H.L. Fast detoxification of drug abuse by acupuncture and electrical stimulation (AES) in combination with naxone. *Comp. Med. East West*, Fall–Winter 1997, 5(3–4): 257–263.
8. Niu, W.M., Liu, H.Y., and Zhang, Y.H. Application of ear acupuncture therapy to treat opium drug abstinence syndrome. *Shang. J. Acupunc. Moxibustion*, 2000, 3(6): 27–29.
9. Avants, S.K. et al. Acupuncture for the treatment of cocaine addiction. Investigation of a needle puncture control. *J. Subst. Abuse*, May–Jun. 12, 1995, 3: 195–205.
10. Marovino, T. Laser auriculotherapy as part of the nicotine detoxification process: evaluation of 1280 subjects and theoretical considerations of a developing model. *Am. J. Acupunc.*, 1994, 22(2): 134.
11. Liu, X.S. Ear point tapping and pressing therapy for giving up smoking in 45 cases. *J. Trad. Chin. Med.*, 1996, 15(1): 33–34.
12. Sun, H. Clinical observation on auricular acupuncture for treatment of pain diseases. *Am. J. Trad. Chin. Med.*, 2001, 2(1): 15–17.

13. Wu, H. et al. Clinical observation and mechanism study in application of auricular-pressing pill for post-operative analgesia. *J. Trad. Chin. Med.*, 1991, 17(1): 26–31.
14. Umeh, B. Ear acupuncture using semi-permanent needles: acceptability, prospects and problems in Nigeria. *Am. J. Acupunc.*, 1988, 16 (1–2): 67–70.
15. Jichova, E., Koenigova, R., and Prusik, K. Acupuncture in patients with thermal injuries. *Act. Chirurgiae. Plasticae.*, 1983, 25(2): 102–108, (in Czech).
16. Lin, J.G., Salahin, H.S., and Lin, J.C. Investigation of the effects of ear acupressure on exercise induced lactic acid levels and the implications for athletic training. *Am. J. Acupunc.*, 1995, 23(4): 309–313.
17. Doubler, F. The treatment of post-polio syndrome with electrostimulation of auricular acupuncture points: an evaluation of twelve patients. *Am. J. Acupunc.*, 1994, 22(1): 15–21.
18. Lewis, G.B.H. An alternative approach to premedication: comparing diazepam with auriculotherapy and a relaxation method. *Am. J. Acupunc.*, Jul.–Sept. 1987, 15(3): 205–214.
19. Wang, S.M. and Kain, Z.N. Auricular acupuncture: a potential treatment for anxiety. *Anesth. Analg.*, Feb. 2001, 92(2): 548–553.
20. Shi, Z.X. Observation of the therapeutic effect of 120 cases of hallucinations treated with auricular acupuncture. *J. Trad. Chin. Med.*, Dec. 1988, 8(4): 263–264.
21. Romoli, M. and Giommi, A. Ear acupuncture in psychosomatic medicine; the importance of the Sanjiao (triple heater) area. *Acupunc. Electrother. Res.*, Jul.–Dec. 1993, 18(3–4): 185–194.
22. Tian, L. Composite acupuncture treatment of mental retardation in children. *J. Trad. Chin. Med.*, Mar. 1995, 15(3): 34–37.
23. Zhang, Y., Li, Y., Tang, X., Ji, C., and Chen, L. The effect of stimulating auricular liver-gall point on the size of a gallbladder of the rabbit. *Zhen Ci Yan Jiu*, 1993 18(1): 73–74, (in Chinese).
24. Gu, X. Clinical study on analgesia for biliary colic with ear acupuncture ear point Erzhong. *Am. J. Acupunc.*, 1993, 21(3): 237–239.
25. Li, Z.Y. et al. Effective observation of 114 cases of cholelithiasis by auricular-plaster therapy. *Chin. Acupunc. Moxibustion*, 1987, 7(5): 23, (in Chinese).
26. Liu, X., Qin, B., and Chen, Y. Observation of the effect of otoacupoint pressure on the motor function of the gallbladder. *J. Trad. Chin. Med.*, Mar. 1993, 13(1): 42.
27. Wang, M.L. Forty-two cases of climacteric syndrome treated with auricular pellet pressure. *J. Trad. Chin. Med.*, Sept. 1991, 11(3): 196–198.
28. Lewers, D., Clelland, J.A., Jackson, J.R., Varner, R.E., and Bergman, J. Transcutaneous electrical nerve stimulation in the relief of primary dysmenorrhea. *Phys. Ther.*, Jan. 1989, 69(1): 3–9.
29. Shapiro, R.S., Christopher, W., and Cicora, B. Effective stimulation of auricular and body acupuncture materials. *Vet. Acupunc. Newsl.*, Jan.–Mar. 1989, 14(1): 25–36.
30. Zhu, B., Wang, Y., and Xu, W. Effect of electroacupuncture on peripheral microcirculation in acute experimental arthritic rats. *Zhen Ci Yan Jiu*, 1993, 18(3): 219–222, (in Chinese).
31. Hep, A., Presek, J., Dolina, J., Ondrowek, L., and Dite, P. Treatment of esophageal motility disorders with acupuncture of the ear (preliminary report), *Unitr. Lek.* Jul. 1995, 41(7): 413–415.

32. Li, F.L., Wang, D., and Ma, X.Y. Treatment of hiccoughs with auricular acupuncture. *J. Trad. Chin. Med.*, 1991, 11(1): 14–16.
33. Zhou, X.Q. and Liu, J.X. Chung-kuo chung hsi I chieh ho tsu chih, Apr. 1993, 13(4): 196, 212–214, (in Chinese).
34. Feng, C. et al. Clinical investigation in cerebral arteriosclerosis treated by acupuncture at auricular Shenmen. *J. Trad. Chin. Med. Alumni*, 2000, 1(1): 11.
35. Zhou, R.X., Zhang, Y.H., et al. Anti-hypertensive effect of auriculo-acupoint pressing therapy – clinical analysis of 274 cases. *J. Trad. Chin. Med.*, 1991, 11(1): 189–192.
36. Huang, H.Q. and Liang, S.Z. Improvement of blood pressure and left cardiac function in patients with hypertension by auricular acupuncture. *Zhong Xi Yi Jie He Za Zhi*, Nov. 1991, 11(11): 643–644, (in Chinese).
37. Gaponiuk, P.I. and Leonova, M.V. The clinical efficacy of auricular electroacupuncture in treating hypertension patients. *Vopr. Kurortol. Fizioter. Lech. Fiz. Kult.*, Jan.–Feb. 1990, 1:13–15, (in Russian).
38. Solun, M.N. and Liaifer, A.L. Acupuncture in the treatment of diabetic angiopathy of the lower extremities. *Probl. Endokrinol. (Mosk.),* Jul.–Aug. 1991, 37(4): 20–23, (in Russian).
39. Chen, L. 408 cases of urinary calculus treated by auriculo-acupoint pressure. *J. Trad. Chin. Med.*, Sept. 1991, 11(3): 193–195.
40. Wang, Q. and Zhao, Y.Y. Treatment of urinary retention due to post-operative anal pain. *J. Trad. Chin. Med.*, Sept. 1991, 11(3): 199–200.
41. Chen, Y.S. and Hu, X.I. Auriculo-acupuncture in 15 cases of discoid lupus erythematosus. *J. Trad. Chin. Med.*, 1985, 5(4): 261–262.
42. Cheng, H.F. Ear point pressure with herbal medicine for treating myopia in youngsters. *Chin. Acupunc. and Moxibustion*, Feb. 1988, 8(1): 22.
43. Liu, H., Lu, Y., Dong, Q., and Zhong, X. Treatment of adolescent myopia by pressure plaster of semen impatientis on otopoints. *J. Trad. Chin. Med.,* Dec. 1991, 14(4): 283–286.
44. Yang, C. et al. 268 cases of myopia treated with injection and pellet pressure at auriculopoints. *J. Trad. Chin. Med.*, Sept. 1993, 13(3): 196–198.

Bibliography

Ackerman, R.W. *The Experience of Women Receiving Auricular Acupuncture Treatment for Chemical Dependency During Pregnancy,* Ph.D. dissertation, The Fielding Institute, Santa Barbara, CA, 1994.

Akhmedov, T.I., Vasil'ev, I.M., and Masliaeva, L.V. The hemodynamic and neurohumoral correlates of the changes in the status of hypertension patients under the influence of acupuncture. *Ter. Arkh.*, 1993, 65(12): 22–24, (in Russian).

Aleksandrina, E.V., Zharkin, A.F., and Gavrilova, A.S. The acupuncture prevention of anomalies in labor strength in pregnant women of a risk group. *Ter. Akush Ginekol.*, (Mosk), 1992, 8–12: 22–24. (in Russian).

Allison, D.B., Kreibich, K., Heshka, S., and Heymsfield, S.B. A randomized placebo-controlled clinical trial of an acupressure device for weight loss. *Int. J. Obes. Related Metab. Disord.*, Sept. 1995, 19(9): 653–658.

Alkaysi, G., Leindler, L., Bajusz, H., and Szarvas, F. The treatment of pathological obesity by a new auricular method: a five year clinical experience. *Am. J. Acupunc.*, 1991, 19(4): 323–328.

Antonio, A.M., Mosiagin, V.V., Iaitskii, N.A., Grinenko, N.N., and Antonova, I.A. The use of auricular puncture in the combined treatment of acute cholecystitis in elderly persons. *Vestn. Khir. IM. I. I. Grek.*, 1995, 154(3): 104–105, (in Russian).

Apostolopoulos, A. Treatment of obesity and weight loss by auricular acupuncture in 800 cases. The Medical Acupuncture Web page. Announced at ICMART, 1996, VII's World Congress, Copenhagen, p. 49.

Asamazova, V.I., Kriukov, A.I., Sako, A.B., Linder, I.B., and Kosiakov, S.I. Study of biologically active currents in endaural ear pharmcophysical intervention. *Vestn. Otorinolaringol.*, Mar.–Apr. 1989, (2): 17–20, (in Russian).

Asamoto, S. and Takeshige, C. Activation of the satiety center by auricular acupuncture point stimulation. *Brain Res. Bull.*, Aug. 1992, 29(2): 157–164.

Avants, S.K. et al. Acupuncture for the treatment of cocaine addiction. Investigation of a needle puncture control. *J. Subst. Abuse*, May–Jun. 1995, 12(3): 195–205.

Avants, S.K., Margolin, A., Holford, T.R., and Kosten, T.R. A randomized controlled trial of auricular acupuncture for cocaine dependence. *Arch. Inter. Med.*, Aug. 2000, 160(15): 2305–2312.

Avants, S.K., Margolin, A., and Kosten, T.R. Cocaine abuse in methadone maintenance programs: integrating pharmacotherapy with psychosocial interventions. *J. Psychoactive Drugs*, 1994, 26(2): 137–146.

Ayyagari, S., Boles, S., Johnson, P., and Lkeber, H. Difficulties in recruiting pregnant substance abusing women into treatment: problems encountered during the Cocaine Alternative Treatment Study (CATS). *Abstr. Book Assoc. Health Ser. Res.*, 1999, 16: 80–81.

Bacek, R. The role of auricular and body acupuncture in nicotine addiction and weight loss. *Deutsche Zeitschrift Fuer. Akupunktur.*, 1986, 29(2): 27–32, (in German).

Bai, Z.H. et al. Ear points in chronic gastritis. *Chin. Acupunc. Moxibustion*, 1986, 6(6): 23–25, (in Chinese).

Ballal, S.G. and Khawaji, Y.N. Auricular stimulation and acupuncture as an adjuvant to an anti-smoking program: analysis of the results of a 1–year experience. *Tuber. Lung Dis.*, Dec. 1992, 73(6): 396.

Baum, J. and Schilling, A.: Combined-electrostimulation-hypalgesia in surgery of the lumbar vertebral column. a tentative evaluation of this method. *Anaesthesist*, May 1979, 28(5): 227–236, (in German).

Ben, H. and Zhu, Y. The effect of electro-acupuncture at auricular and body acupoints on the curve changes of the pressure-volume of urinary bladder and the electric activity of pelvic nerves of rat. *Zhen Ci Yan Jiu*, 1995, 20(2): 51–54, (in Chinese).

Bobrov, O.E., Radzikhovskii, A.P., Loboda, D.I., Ogorodnik, P.V., Chmel, V.B., and Ligonenko, A.V. Several problems of surgical treatment in acute biliary pancreatitis. *Klin. Khir.*, 1991, 5: 20–23.

Bondi, N. and Albo, R. Dysmenorrhea, acupuncture treatment of 40 cases coming to our attention. *Minerva Med.*, Sept. 1981, 15: 72(33): 2227–2230, (in Italian).

Boscq, C. Abord dela problematique alcoolique a partir d'un lieu de soins. *Rev. Fr. Acupunc.*, 1994, 20(78): 10–15, (in French).

Bragin, E.O. Alteration of opiate-like substance content in auricular electroacupuncture analgesia of rats. *Voprosy. Medit. Khimii.*, 1982, 28(4): 102–105, (in Russian).

Brewington, V., Smith, M., and Lipton, D. Acupuncture as a detoxification treatment: an analysis of controlled research. *J. Subst. Abuse Treat.*, Jul.–Aug. 1994, 11(4): 289–307.

Brigo, B. and Campacci, R. Antismoking treatment by needle puncture of the ear. *Riabilitazione*, 1980, 13(4): 191–197, (in Italian).

Brumbaugh, A.G. Acupuncture: new perspectives in chemical dependency treatment. *J. Subst. Abuse Treat.*, Jan.–Feb. 1993, 10(1): 35–43.

Brumbaugh, A.G. *Transformation and Recovery: A Guide for the Design and Development of Acupuncture–Based Chemical Dependency Treatment Programs*. Stillpoint Press, New York, 1993.

Brumbaugh, A.G. *Acupuncture for Withdrawal Management and Stabilization: Successful Conceptual Foundation for Program Retention and Positive Outcomes in Chemical Dependency.*, Stillpoint Press, New York, 1998, p. 3.

Bullock, M.L. et al. Controlled trial of acupuncture for severe recidivist alcoholism. *Lancet*, 1989, 1:1435.

Bullock, M.L., Kiresuk, T.J., Pheley, A.M., Culliton, P.D., and Lenz, S.K. Auricular acupuncture in the treatment of cocaine abuse. A study of efficacy and dosing. *J. Subst. Abuse Treat.*, Jan. 1999, 16(1): 31–38.

Bullock, M.L., Umen, A.J., Culliton, P.D., and Olander, R.T. Acupuncture treatment of alcoholic recidivism: A pilot study. *Am. J. Acupunc.*, 1987, 15(4): 313–320.

Boureau, F. and Willer J.C. Failure of naloxone to modify the anti-tobacco effect of acupuncture (author's transl). *Nouv. Presse Med.*, Apr. 22, 1978, 7(16): 1401, (in French).

Ceccherelli, F., Ambrosio, F., Adami, M.G. et al. Failure of high frequency auricular electrical stimulation to relieve postoperative pain after cholecystectomy. Results not improved by administration of aprotinin. *Dtsch. Z. Akupunktur.*, 1985, 28(4): 87–92, (in German).

Ceccherelli, F., Manai, G., Ambrosio, F., Angel, A., Valenti, S., Facco, E., and Giron, G.P. Influence of acupuncture on the postoperative complications following ketamine anesthesia. The importance of manual stimulation of point R and shenmen. *Acupunc. Electrother. Res.*, 1981, 6(4): 255–264.

Chandnani, J.K. The treatment of obesity with acupuncture. *WFAS 1st Conf.* (Eng.), 1987.

Chen, C., Li, Y.F., and Zhong, C. Treatment of 30 cases of migraine by combination of Lu's compound acupuncture techniques and auricular application. TCM Shang. *J.Acupunc. Moxibustion*, 2001, 4(3): 52–53.

Chen, G. Advances in researches in auriculo-acupoints. *J. Trad. Chin. Med.*, 1991, 11(3): 216–233.

Chen, G. et al. How to enhance the therapeutic efficacy of auriculo-point seed pressing method in the treatment of cholecystitis. *J. Trad. Chin. Med.*, 1991, 11(4): 263–271.

Chen, G.S. Enkephalin, drug addiction and acupuncture. *Am. J. Chin. Med.*, 1977, 5(1): 25–30.

Chen, J.Y.P. Treatment of cigarette smoking by auricular acupuncture: a report of 184 cases. *Am. J. Acupunc.*, 1979, 7(3): 229–234.

Chen, K. Treatment of headache with traditional auriculoacupoint therapy. *J. Trad. Chin. Med.*, 1993 Sept., 13(3): 230–233.

Chen, L. 408 cases of urinary calculus treated by auriculo-acupoint pressure. *J. Trad. Chin. Med.*, Sept. 1991, 11(3): 193–195.

Chen, M.C. 112 cases of juvenile myopia treatment by auricular acupressure. *J. Trad. Chin. Med.*, Sept. 1989, 9(3): 173.

Chen. S, Therapeutic effects of ear acupuncture in 52 cases with reaction to blood transfusion or fluid infusion. *World J. Acupunc. Moxibustion*, 1995, 5(2): 26–28.

Chen, Z. Acupuncture treatment of headache. *J. Trad. Chin. Med.*, Dec. 1994, 14(4): 272–275.

Chen, Z. Treatment of ulcerative colitis with acupuncture. *J. Trad. Chin. Med.*, Sept. 1995, 15(3): 231–233.

Chen, Z. Acupuncture treatment for gastroptosis. *J. Trad. Chin. Med.*, Dec. 1996, 16(4): 3034–3036.

Chen, Y.S. and Hu, X.I. Auriculo-acupuncture in 15 cases of discoid lupus erythematosus. *J. Trad. Chin. Med.*, 1985, 5(4): 261–262.

Cheng, H.F. Ear point pressure with herbal medicine for treating myopia in youngsters. *Chin. Acupunc. Moxibustion,* Feb. 1988, 8(1): 22.

Cheng, R.S., Pomeranz, B., and Yu, G. Electroacupuncture treatment of morphine-dependent mice reduces signs of withdrawal, without showing cross-tolerance. *Eur. J. Pharmacol.,* Dec. 1980, 1968(4): 477–481.

Cheung, C.K.T. The treatment of cigarette smoking by electro-acupuncture, intradermal needle, and diet precautions. *Brit. J. Acupunc.,* 1986; 9(1): 26–28.

China Association of Acupuncture and Moxibustion. Selections for Articles Abstracts on Acupuncture and Moxibustion. Beijing, China, 1987.

Choy, Y.M., Tso, W.W., Fung, K.P., Leung, K.C., Tsang, Y.F., Lee, L.Y., and Tsang, D. Suppression of narcotic withdrawals and plasma ACTH by auricular electroacupuncture. *Biochem. Biophys. Res. Comm.,* May 1, 1978, 82(1): 305–309.

Chirstensen, A. EAP and post-operative pain. *Am. J. Acupunc.,* 1989, 17: 269.

Chun, S. and Heather, A.J. Auriculotherapy: microcurrent application on the external ear – clinical analysis of a pilot study on 57 chronic pain syndromes. *Am. J. Chin. Med.,* 1974, 2(4): 399–405.

Clavel, F., Benhamou, S., and Flamant, R. Nicotine dependence and secondary effects of smoking cessation. *J. Behav. Med.,* 1987, 10(6): 555–558.

Clavel, F. and Benhamou, S. Tobacco withdrawal. Comparison of the efficacy of various methods. Intermediate results of a comparative study. *Press Med.,* Apr. 14, 1984, 13(16): 975–977, (in French).

Clavel, F. and Paoletti, C. A study of various smoking cessation programs based on close to 1000 volunteers recruited from the general population: 1–month results. *Rev. Epidemiol. Sante Publique.,* 1990, 38(2): 133–138, (in French).

Clavel–Chapelon, F., Paoletti, C., and Benhamou, S. Smoking cessation rates 4 years after treatment by nicotine gum and acupuncture. *Prev. Med.,* Jan.–Feb. 1997, 26(1): 25–28.

Clavel–Chapelon, F., Paoletti, C., and Benhanou, S. A randomized 2x2 factorial design to evaluate different smoking cessation methods. *Rev. Epidemiol. Sante Publique.,* 1992, 40(3): 187–190.

Clement–Jones, V., McLoughlin, L., Lowry, P.J., et al. Acupuncture in heroin addicts: changes in net-enkephalin and endorphin in blood and cerebrospinal fluid. *Lancet*, 1979, 2(8139): 380–382.

Cocchi, R., Lorini, G., Fusari, A., and Carrossino, R. Experience with detoxification and weaning of heroin addicts by means of acupuncture, gabergic drugs and psychopharmacologic agents in low doses. *Minerva Med.,* May 19, 1979, 70(24): 1735–1744, (in Italian).

Coleman, T. Acupuncture in smoking cessation. *Brit. J. Gen. Pract.,* Nov. 1998, (436): 1789.

Cottraux, J., Schbath, J., Messy, P., Mollard, E., Juenet, C., and Collet, L. Predictive value of MMPI scales on smoking cessation programs outcomes. *Acta Psychiatr. Belg.,* Jul.–Aug. 1986, 86(4): 463–469 (in Belgian).

Cottraux, J.A., Harf, R., Boissel, J.P., Schbath, J., Bouvard, M., and Gillet, J. Smoking cessation with behavior therapy of acupuncture — a controlled study. *Behav. Res. Ther.*, 1983, 21(4): 417–424.

Cox, B.C. Patient motivation: a factor in weight reduction with auriculo– acupuncture. *Am. J. Acupunc.*, 1975, 3(4): 339–341.

Craver, F., Benhamou, S., Company–Huertas, A., and Flamant, R. Helping people to stop smoking: randomized comparison of groups being treated with acupuncture and nicotine gum with control group. *Brit. Med. J.* (Clin. Res. ed.), Nov. 30, 1985, 291(6508): 1538–1539.

Cui, M. Advances in studies on acupuncture abstinence. *J. Trad. Chin. Med.*, Mar. 1996, 16(1): 65–69.

Cui, S.G., Xu, Z.Z., and Zhang, F.S. Obesity treated by ear acupuncture. *Chin. Acupunc. Moxibustion*, 1987, 7(1): 17.

Culliton, P.D. and Kiresuk, T.J. Overview of substance abuse acupuncture treatment research. *J. Altern. Complement. Med.*, Spring 1996, 2(1): 149–165.

Dai, G. Advances in the acupuncture treatment of acne. *J. Trad. Chin. Med.*, Mar. 1997, 17(1): 65–72.

Dale, R.A. Addictions and acupuncture: The treatment methods, formulae, effectiveness, and limitations. *Am. J. Acupunc.*, 1993, 21(3): 247–266.

Deng, D.Y. Ear acupuncture in the treatment of hepatolithiasis. *Am. J. Acupunc.*, 1986, 14: 274.

Deung, C.Y. and Spoerel, W.E. Effect of auricular acupuncture on pain. *Am. J. Clin. Med.*, 1974, 2(2): 247–260.

Dolgikh, V.G. and Reshetniak, V.K. Changes in the jaw-opening reflex during anesthesia resulting from auricular stimulation. *Biull. Eksp. Biol. Med.*, May 1987, 103(5): 520–521, (in Russian).

Dong, S.R. Clinical analysis of therapeutic efficiency in 365 cases of cholelithiasis treated by pressure. *Am. J. Acupunc.*, 1986, 14: 273.

Dong , A.Q. Uses of auricular acupoint needle imbedding therapy to stop smoking. *Chin. Acupunc. Moxibustion*, 1985, 5(4): 47–48.

Doubler, F. The treatment of post-polio syndrome with electrostimulation of auricular acupuncture points: an evaluation of twelve patients. *Am. J. Acupunc.*, 1994, 22(1): 15–21.

Duan, R.L., Shen, Z.B., and Liu, X.D. Obesity treated by auricular acupoint pressure. Analysis of 200 cases. Shanghai *J. Chin. Trad. Med.*, 1986, 7(5): 215.

Dung, H.C. Acupuncture points of the cervical plexus. *Am. J. Chin. Med.*, Summer 1984, 12(1–4): 94–105.

Dung, H.C. Clinical experiences in using acupuncture to help smoking withdrawal. *Int. J. Chin. Med.*, 1986, 3(1): 5–16.

Dung, H.C. Attempts to reduce body weight through auricular acupuncture. *Am. J. Acupunc.*, 1986, 14(2): 117–122.

Ercolani, M., Zusshini, G.E., and Poli, E.G. Acupuncture, auriculotherapy and craniopuncture in the treatment of functional amblyopia in children. *Minerva Med.*, Nov. 3, 1983, 74(42): 2537–2540, (in Italian).

Facco, E., Manani, G., Angel, A., Vincenti, E., Tambuscio, B., Ceccherelli, F., Troletti, G., Ambrosio, F., and Giron, G.P. Comparison study between acupuncture and pentazocine analgesic and respiratory post-operative effects. *Am. J. Chin. Med.*, Autumn 1981, 9(3): 225–235.

Fang, Y.A., Li, Q.S., and Zhang, Q.S. Relation between gustatory sense and plasma enkephalin during withdrawal of smoking addiction by auricular acupuncture. *Shanghai J. Acupunc. Moxibustion*, 1985, (3): 1–3.

Feng, C. et al. Clinical investigation in cerebral arteriosclerosis treated by acupuncture at auricular *Shenmen*. *J. Trad. Chin. Med.* Alumni., 2000, 1(1): 11.

Fong, K. Bronchial-asthma treated by He–Ne laser radiation on ear points. *Chin. J. Acupunc. Moxibustion*, 1990, 3(4): 272–273.

Freibott, A. Ambulatory acupuncture assisted drug withdrawal program in Frankfurt an Main. A pilot experiment. *AKU*, 1995, 23(3): 176–180, (in German).

Friedmaan, J. Auricular acupuncture for smoking. *Acupunc. Electrother. Res.*, 1992, 17(2): 149–150.

Fuller, J.A. Smoking withdrawal and acupuncture. *Med. J. Aust.*, Jan. 9, 1982, 1(1): 28–29.

Gaa'l, C.L. and Freebain, C. Ear acupuncture relaxation therapy in alcoholics. *Med. J. Aust.*, 1979, 2(4): 179–180.

Gandhi, R. The uses of auricular acupuncture in the field of substance misuse. *Psychiatr. Care*, 1996, 3 (Suppl. 1): 40–41.

Gapionuk, P.I. and Leonova, M.V. The clinical efficacy of auricular electroacupuncture in treating hypertension patients. *Vopr. Kurortol. Fizioter. Lech. Fiz. Kult.*, Jan.–Feb. 1990, 1: 13–15, (in Russian).

Gaponiuk, P.I., Leonova, M.V., Sherkovina, T.I., and Iotova, V.G. The effect of auricular electroacupuncture on the initial manifestations of cerebral circulatory failure in hypertension patients. *Vopr. Kurortol. Fizioter. Lech. Fiz. Kult.*, Nov.–Dec. 1990, 6: 31–34, (in Russian).

Gaponiuk, P.I., Sherkovina, T.I., and Leonova, M.V. Acupuncture stimulation of the auricular points in hypertension patients with hypo– and eukinetic types of blood circulation. *Vopr. Kurortol. Fizioter. Lech. Fiz. Kult.*, Jul.–Aug. 1987, 4: 53–54, (in Russian).

Gerhard, I. and Postneek, F. Auricular acupuncture in the treatment of female infertility, *Gynecolog. Endocrinol.*, 1992, 6(3): 171.

Gerhard, I. and Postneek, F. Possibilities of therapy by ear acupuncture in female sterility. *Geburtshilfe Frauenheilkd.*, Mar. 1988, 48(3): 165–171, (in German).

Gersdorgg, M. and Robillard, T. Treatment of tinnitus by electrical simulation of the ear. *Acta Otohinolaryngol. Be lg.*, 1985, 39(3): 583–612, (in French).

Giglio, J.C. A randomized controlled trial of auricular acupuncture for cocaine dependence: treatments vs. outcomes. *Arch. Intern. Med.*, Mar. 26, 2001, 161(6): 894–895.

Gilbey, V. and Neumann, B. Auricular acupuncture for smoking withdrawal. *Am. J. Acupunc.*, Jul.–Sept. 1997, 5(3): 239–247.

Gillams, J., Lewith, G.T., and Machin, D. Acupuncture and group therapy in stopping smoking. *Practitioner*, Mar. 1984, 228(1389): 341–344.

Giller, R.M. Auricular acupuncture and weight reduction; a control study. *Am. J. Acupunc.*, 1975, 3(2): 151–153.

Gofman, S.S. The treatment of occupational fluorosis by acupuncture reflexotherapy. *Gig. Tr. Prof. Zabol.*, 1991, 11: 40–42, (in Russian).

Goidenko, V.S., Perminova, I.S., and Sitel, A.B. Use of auricular acupuncture reflexotherapy in treating Sjogren's disease. *Stomatologiia (Mosk).*, Jul.–Aug. 1985, 64(4): 47–48, (in Russian).

Gong, C.M. New effective alcohol abstinence acupuncture treatment. *Am. J. Acupunc.*, 1988, 16: 181.

Greene, H.L., Goldberg, R.J., and Ockene, J.K. Cigarette smoking: the physician's role in cessation and maintenance. *J. Gen. Intern. Med.*, 1988, 3(1): 75–78.

Greenwood, M. The use of ear acupuncture to promote vaginal delivery after cesarean section. *Am. J. Acupunc.*, 1992, 20 (4): 305–312.

Groblas, A. Auricular acupuncture and obesity. *Shanghai J. Acupunc. Moxibustion*, 1984, 2: 43–44.

Gu, X. Clinical study on analgesia for biliary colic with ear acupuncture ear point *Erzhong. Am. J. Acupunc.*, 1993, 21(3): 237–239.

Gu, Y. et al. Observation of 473 cases of weight reduction treated by implanting seeds at ear points. *Chin. Acupunc. Moxibustion*, 1988, 8(1); 15–16.

Gu, Y.S. Clinical observation on weight reduction by pressing auricular points with semen vaccariae: a report of 473 cases. *J. Trad. Chin. Med.*, Sept. 1989, 9(3): 166.

Gurevich, M.I. et al. Is auricular acupuncture beneficial in the inpatient treatment of substance abusing patients? A pilot study. *J. Subst. Abuse Treat.*, Mar.–Apr. 1996, 13(2): 165–171.

Haegele, P.A. 20 years of experience in detoxification and withdrawal treatment with acupuncture. *AKU*, 1995, 23(3): 171–175, (in German).

He, D., Berg, J.E., and Hostmark, A.T. Effects of acupuncture on smoking cessation or reduction for motivated smokers. *Prev. Med.*, 1997, 26(2): 208–214.

Heimer, H. and Muller, S.K. Acupuncture as after care following injuries of the upper extremities. *Handchirurgie*, 1977, 9(3): 129–143, (in German).

Huang, M.H., Yang, R.C., and Hu, S.H. Preliminary results of triple therapy for obesity: a clinical observation of 39 cases. *Int. J. Obes. Related Metab. Disord.*, 1996, 20(9): 830–836.

Huang, H.Q. and Liang, S.Z. Improvement of blood pressure and left cardiac function in patients with hypertension by auricular acupuncture. *Zhong Xi Yi Jie He Za Zhi*, Nov. 1991, 11(11): 643–644, (in Chinese).

Ivanov, V.A. and Iakovleva, E.A. Auricular reflexotherapy of humeroscapular periarthritis. *Ortop. Travmatol. Protez.*, Sept. 1986, 9: 44–45, (in Russian).

Jensen, L.B., Melsen, B., and Jensen, S.B. Effect of acupuncture on headache measured by reduction in number of attacks and use of drugs. *Scand. J. Dent. Res.*, Oct. 1979, 87(5): 373–380.

Jerner, B., Skogh, M., and Vahlquist, A. A controlled trial of acupuncture in psoriasis; no convincing effect. *Acta Derm. Venereol.*, 1997, 77(2): 154–156, (in Norwegian).

Ji, Y. 776 cases of pain treated with auriculopressure therapy. *J. Trad. Chin. Med.*, Dec. 1992, 12(4): 275–276.

Jiang, A. and Cui, M. Analysis of therapeutic effects of acupuncture on abstinence from smoking. *J. Trad. Chin. Med.*, Mar. 1994, 14(1): 56–63.

Jiang, H. Ear acupuncture for hypotonia in gastrointestinal examination. *AJR Am. J. Roentgeneol.*, Oct. 1986, 147(4): 862.

Jiang, Y.G. et al. Effect of EAP on gastric motility in rats. *AJA, (Abstract)*, 1987, 15: 372, ex *Gastroenterology*, 1987, 92: 1454.

Jiang, Y.S. Body needling combined with auricular acupuncture to stop smoking. Report of 10 cases. *Sichuan Trad. Chin. Med.*, 1986, 4(65): 54, (in Chinese).

Jichova, E., Koenigova, R., and Prusik, K. Acupuncture in patients with thermal injuries. *Acta Chirurgiae. Plasticae.*, 1983, 25(2): 102–108, (in Chinese).

Jin, Y., Wu, L., and Xia, Y. Clinical study on painless labor under drugs combined with acupuncture analgesia. *Zhen Ci Yan Jiu*, 1996, 21(3): 9–17, (in Chinese).

Ju, X.S. Auricular electroacupuncture for withdrawal of smoking addiction. Analysis of 89 cases. *Shanghai J. Acupunc. Moxibustion*, 1985, (2): 9.

Kenyon, J.N., Knight, C.J., and Wells, C. Randomised double-blind trial on the immediate effects of naloxone on classical Chinese acupuncture therapy for chronic pain. *Acupunc. Electrother. Res.*, 1983, 8(1): 17–24.

Kitsenko, V.P. and Zaikina, T.A. Comprehensive treatment of cochlear neuritis using auricular reflexotherapy on an outpatient basis. *Vest. Otorinlaringol.*, May–Jun. 1979, 3: 62–63. (in Russian).

Konefal, J. et al. The impact of the addition of an acupuncture treatment program to an existing Metro–Dade County outpatient substance abuse treatment facility. *J. Addict. Dis.*, 1994, 13(3): 71–99.

Konefal, J., Duncan, R., and Clemence, C. Comparison of three levels of auricular acupuncture in an outpatient substance abuse program. *Altern. Med. J.*, 1995, 2(5): 8–17.

Koskenniemi, T. Effect of ear acupuncture for obesity. *Acupunc. Electrother. Res.*, 1985, 10(3): 231.

Krause, A.W., Clelland, J.A., Knowles, C.J., and Jackson, J.R. Effects of unilateral and bilateral auricular transcutaneous electrical nerve stimulation on cutaneous pain threshold. *Phys Ther.*, Apr. 1987, 67(4): 507–511.

Kroenig, R.J. and Oleson, T.F. Rapid narcotic detoxification in chronic pain patients treated with auricular acupuncture and naloxone. *Int. J. Addict.*, 1985, 20(9): 1347–1360.

Kruger, H. and Kruger, P. Ear acupuncture in motor disorders of small animals. *Prakt. Tierarzt.*, 1980, 61: 119–129, (in German).

Kubista, E., Boschitsch, E., and Spona, J. Effect of ear-acupuncture on the LH–concentration in serum in patients with secondary amenorrhea (author's transl.). *Wein. Med. Wochenschr.*, Mar. 15, 1981, 131(5): 123–126, (in German).

Kusumi, Y.T. New approach to smoking cessation with ear acupuncture and behavior modification therapy. *Am. J. Acupunc.*, 1986, 14(4): 325–332.

Lacroix, J.C. and Besancon, F. Tobacco withdrawal. Efficacy of acupuncture in a comparative trial. *Ann. Med. Interne.* (Paris), Apr. 1977, 128(4): 405–408, (in French).

Lagrue, G., Pouopy, J.L., Grillot, A., and Ansquer, J.C. Antismoking acupuncture. Short-term results of a double-blind comparative study (letter). *Nouv. Presse Med.*, Mar. 15, 1980, 9(13): 966, (in French).

Lao, H.H. A retrospective study on the use of acupuncture for the prevention of alcoholic recidivism. *Am. J. Acupunc.*, 1995, 23(1): 29–33.

Lapeer, G.L. Trigeminal neuralgia: treatment failure with auriculotherapy: two case reports. *Cranio*, Jan. 1990, 8(1): 55–59.

Lapeer, G.L. Auriculotherapy in dentistry. *Cranio*, July 1986, 4(3): 266–275.

Lau, H.B., Wang, B., and Wong, S.D. Effect of acupuncture on weight reduction. Am, *J. Acupunc.*, 1975, 3(4): 335–338.

Lau, M.P. Acupuncture and addiction: an overview. *Addict. Dis.*, 1976, 2(3): 449–463.

Law, M. and Tang, J.L. People stop smoking. *Arch. Intern. Med.*, Oct. 9, 1995, 155(18): 1933–1941.

Lebeau, B., Vidal, C., Billion, A., Torcy, M., and Rochemaure, J. Tobacco detoxification with acupuncture and group psychotherapy. *Rev. Med. Interne.*, Nov. 1986, 7(5): 471–476, (in French).

Lei, Z.P. Acupuncture in the treatment of obesity. Analysis of 42 cases. *J. Trad. Chin. Med.*, 1987, 28(5): 5203.

Lei, Z.Q. Stop smoking by auricular acupuncture. A case report. *Shaanxi Corres. J. Trad. Chin. Med.*, 1989, (3): 19.

Lequang, T., Badaoui, R., Riboulot, M., Verhaighe, P., and Ossart, M. Postoperative analgesia by auriculotherapy during laparoscopic cholecystectomy. *Cah. Anesthesiol.*, 1996, 44(4): 289–292, (in French).

Leung, A.S.H. Acupuncture treatment of withdrawal symptoms. *Am. J. Acupunc.*, 1977, 5(1): 3–50.

Leung, J.P. Smoking cessation by auricular acupuncture and behavioral therapy. *Psychologia*, Sept. 1991, 34(3): 177–187.

Leung, CY. and Spoerel, W.R. Effect of auricular acupuncture on pain. *Am. J. Chin. Med.*, 1974, 2(3): 247–260.

Lewenberg, A. Electroacupuncture and antidepressant treatment of alcoholism in a private practice. *Clin. Ther.*, 1985, 7(5): 611–617.

Lewenberg, A. The utility of acupuncture in combination with antidepressants or clonidine in the treatment of opiate addiction. *Adv. Ther.*, 1985, 2 (4): 143–149.

Lewers, D., Clelland, J.A., Jackson, J.R., Varner, R.E., and Bergman, *J.* Transcutaneous electrical nerve stimulation in the relief of primary dysmenorrhea. *Phys. Ther.*, Jan. 1989, 69(1): 3–9.

Lewis, G.B.H. An alternative approach to premedication: comparing diazepam with auriculotherapy and a relaxation method. *Am. J. Acupunc.*, Jul.–Sept. 1987, 15(3): 205–214.

Lewis, S.M., Clelland, J.A., Knowles, C.J., Jackson, J.R., and Dimick, A.R. Effects of auricular acupuncture-like transcutaneous electric nerve stimulation on pain levels following wound care in patients with burns: a pilot study. *J. Burn Care Rehabil.*, Jul.–Aug. 1990, 11(4): 322–329.

Lewith, G.T., Field, J., and Machin, D. Acupuncture compared with placebo in post-herpetic pain. *Pain*, Dec. 1983, 17(4): 361–368.

Lewith, G. The treatment of tobacco addiction. *Compl. Ther. Med.*, July 1995, 3(3): 142–145.

Li, B.N. Stop smoking by intradermal needle imbedding method at auricular acupoints. *Chin. Acupunc. Moxibustion*, 1986, 6(5): 7.

Li, B.N. Quit smoking with ear acupuncture in 27 cases. *J. Chin. Acupunc. Moxibustion*, 1988, 1(3–4): 61.

Li, F.L. and Wang, D. Treatment of hiccoughs with auriculoacupuncture. *J. Trad. Chin. Med.*, 1991, 11(1): 14–16.

Li, J.Q. Chronic pyogenic otitis media treated by Ear–AP. *Am. J. Acupunc.*, 1986, 14: 68.

Li, W.A. 439 cases of myopia in adolescence treated by embedding needles at ear acupoints. *Chin. J. Acupunc. Moxibustion*, 1991; 4(2): 115–116.

Li, L. Application of acupuncture anaesthesia in cystoscopy. *J. Trad. Chin. Med.*, Mar. 1994, 14(1): 30–31.

Li, Q.S., Liu, Z.Y., Ma, H.J., Lu, Y.Y., Fang, Y.A., Hou, Y.Z., Cao, S.H., and Zhang, Z.H. A preliminary study on the mechanism of ear-acupuncture for withdrawal of smoking. *J. Trad. Chin. Med.*, Dec. 1987, 7(4): 243–247.

Li, Q.S., Cao, S.H., Xie, G.M., Gan, Y.H., Ma, H.J., Lu, J.Z., and Zhang, Z.H. Combined traditional Chinese medicine and Western medicine. Relieving effects of Chinese herbs, ear-acupuncture and epidural morphine on postoperative pain in liver cancer. *Chin. Med. J.* (Eng.)., Apr. 1994, 107(4): 289–294.

Li, X. Treatment of hiccough with auriculo-acupuncture and auriculo-pressure – a report of 85 cases. *J. Trad. Chin. Med.*, Dec. 1990, 10(4): 257–259.

Li, Y. Treatment of 86 cases of facial spasm by acupuncture and pressure on otopoints. *J. Trad. Chin. Med.*, Mar. 2000, 20(1): 3–5.

Li, Y., Tang, X., Zhang, Y., and Wu, F. The effect of stimulating the auricular liver-gall acupoint with electrode on synaptic on nucleus originis dorsalis nervi vagi in rabbits. *Zhen Ci Yan Jiu*, 1992, 17(3): 201–206, (in Chinese).

Li, Z.Y. et al. Effective observation of 114 cases of cholelithiasis by auricular-plaster therapy. *Chin. Acupunc. Moxibustion,* 1987, 7(5): 23, (in Chinese).

Lia, H., Lu, Y., and Dong, Q. Treatment of adolescent myopia by pressure plaster of semen inpatientis on otopoints. *J. Trad. Chin. Med.*, Dec. 1994, 14(4): 282.

Lian, N. Insomnia treated by auricular pressing therapy. *J. Trad. Chin. Med.*, Sept. 1990, 10(3): 174–175.

Liang, S.J. Obesity treated by auricular acupoint pressure with semen vaccariae segetalis. *Chin. Acupunc. Moxibustion,* 1985, 5(6): 28.

Liao, T.J., Nakanishi, H., and Nishikawa, H. The effect of acupuncture stimulation of the middle latency auditory evoked potential. *Tohoku J. Exp. Med.*, Jun. 1993, 170(2): 103–112, (in Japanese).

Lin, J.G., Salahin, H.S., and Lin, J.C. Investigation of the effects of ear acupressure on exercise induced lactic acid levels and the implications for athletic training. *Am. J. Acupunc.*, 1995, 23(4): 309–313.

Lipton, D.S. et al. Acupuncture for crack-cocaine detoxification: experimental evaluation of efficacy. *J. Subst. Abuse.*, May–Jun. 1994, 11(3): 205–215.

Liqun, Z. How to promote the therapeutic effect of auriculotherapy in the treatment of vascular hypertension. *J. Trad. Chin. Med.*, Sept. 1995, 50: 37.

Liu, G. 215 cases of obesity treated with TCM modalities. *J. Trad. Chin. Med.*, Jun. 1993, 13(2): 97–100.

Liu, H., Lu, Y., Dong, Q., and Zhong, X. Treatment of adolescent myopia by pressure plaster of semen impatientis on otopoints. *J. Trad. Chin. Med.*, Dec. 1991, 14(4): 283–286.

Liu, H.H. Obesity treated by ear point embedding. Clinical analysis of 567 cases. *Shanghai J. Acupunc. Moxibustion*, 1986, 5(4): 22.

Liu, J. Effects of acupuncture on myoelectric activity of Oddi's sphincter in humans. *J. Trad. Chin. Med.*, Sept. 1993, 13(3): 189–190.

Liu, X., Qin, B., and Chen, Y. Observation of the effect of otoacupoint pressure on the motor function of the gall bladder. *J. Trad. Chin. Med.*, Mar. 1993, 13(1): 42.

Liu, X., Qin, B., and Chen, Y. Observation on the treatment of 393 cases of obesity by semen pressure on auricular points. *J. Trad. Chin. Med.*, Mar. 1993, 13(1): 27–30.

Liu, X.L. et al. Analysis of the therapeutic effect of 548 cases of infantile trachitis treated with ear pressure method. *Chin. Acupunc. Moxibustion,* Oct. 1998, 8(5): 15–16.

Liu, X.S. Ear point tapping and pressing therapy for giving up smoking in 45 cases. *J. Trad. Chin. Med.*, 1996, 15(1): 33–34.

Liu, Y. Experimental study of electro-acupuncture on auditory impairment caused by kanamycin in guinea pigs. *J. Trad. Chin. Med.*, Mar. 1999, 19(1): 59–64.

Liu, Z., Sun, F., Li, J., Han, Y., Wei, Q., and Liu, C. Application of acupuncture and moxibustion for keeping shape. *J. Trad. Chin. Med.*, Dec. 1988, 18(4): 265–271.

Liu, Z. Effect of acupuncture and moxibustion on the high density lipoprotein cholesterol in simple obesity. *Zhen Ci Yan Jiu*, 1990, 15: 227–231, (in Chinese).

Liu, Z. Recent progress in studies on weight reduction by acupuncture and moxibustion. *J. Trad. Chin. Med.*, Sept. 1995, 15(3): 224–230.

Lomontagne, Y., Annable, L., and Gagnon, M.A. Acupuncture for smokers: lack of long-term therapeutic effect in a controlled study. *Can. Med. Assoc. J.*, Apr. 5 1980, 122(7): 787–790.

Long, W., Zhang, N., and Zhang, Q.M. Auricular sticking therapy of obesity. Report of 72 cases. *J. Gansu. Coll. Trad. Chin. Med.*, 1989, 3: 49–50.

Longobardi, A.G., Clelland, J.A., Knowles, C.J., and Jackson, J.R. Effects of auricular transcutaneous electrical nerve stimulation on distal extremity pain: a pilot study. *Phys. Ther.*, Jan. 1989, 69: 10–17.

Low, S.A. Acupuncture and nicotine withdrawal. *Med. J. Aust.*, Nov. 12, 1977, 2(20): 687.

Low, S.A. Letter. Acupuncture and heroin withdrawal. *Med. J. Aust.*, Aug. 31, 1974, 2(9): 341.

Lowe, L. *A Focus on Acupuncture Research*, presented by the California Department of Corrections at the 5th annual conference of the National Acupuncture Detoxification Associatoin, March 1994, San Francisco.

Lu, M.Z., Zhou, K.Y., and Li, Z.Z. Auricular acupoint pressure therapy for obesity. Analysis of 1000 cases. *Guizhou. Med. J.*, 1986, 10(5): 6–7, (in Chinese).

Lu, Z. and Chey, W.Y. EAP stimulates non-parietal cell secretion of the stomach in dogs. *Am. J. Acupunc.*, 1984, (Abs.) 12: 278, ex *Life Sci.*, 1984, 34: 2233–2238.

Lu, Z.C. and Yang, Y.F. Auricular point sticking therapy of simple obesity – changes in blood lipids and lipoproteins in 29 cases. *Nanjing Coll. Trad. Chi. Med.*, 1989, 2: 40.

Luo, Y.F. Stop smoking by needle embedding at auricular acupoints and oral administration of Chinese herbal drug. *Sichuan J. Trad. Chin. Med.*, 1988, 6(5), (in Chinese).

Lubbe, A.M. Auriculotherapy in canine thoracolumbar disc disease. *J. S. Afr. Vet. Assoc.*, Dec. 1990, 61(4): 187.

Lun, X. and Rong, L. Twenty-five cases of intractable cutaneous pruritus treated by auricular acupuncture. *J. Trad. Chin. Med.*, Dec. 2000, 20(4): 287–288.

Lyrenas, S. et al. AP and EAP in the treatment of focal scleroderma, *Am. J. Acupunc.*, (Abst.) 1988, 16:269, ex *Gynaecol. Obstetr. Invest.*, 1987, 24: 217–224.

Mahomedy, Y.M. Therapeutic application of organ electrodermal diagnostics for pain. *S. Afr. Med. J.*, May 1998, 88(5): 577–578.

Man, P.L. and Chuang, M.Y. Acupuncture in methadone withdrawal. *Int. J. Addict.*, Aug. 1980, 15(6): 921–926.

Marcus, P. The withdrawal of habituating substances. *Acupunc. Med.*, Nov. 1993, 11(2): 76–79.

Margolin, A., Avants, S.K., Birch, S., Falk, C.X., and Kleber, H.D. Methodological investigations for a multisite trial of auricular acupuncture for cocaine addiction: a study of active and control auricular zones. *J. Subst. Abuse Treat.*, Nov.–Dec. 1996, 13(6): 471–481.

Margolin, A., Avants, S.K., Chang, P., and Kosten, T.R. Cocaine abuse in methadone maintenance programs: integrating pharmacotherapy with psychosocial interventions. *J. Psychoact. Drugs*, 1994, 26(2): 137–146.

Margolin, A., Avants, S.K., Birch, S., Falk, C.X., and Kleber, H.D. Methodological investigations for a multisite trial of auricular acupuncture for cocaine addiction: a study of active and control auricular zones. *J. Subst. Abuse Treat.*, Nov.–Dec. 1996, 13(6): 471–481.

Margolin, A., Avants, S.K., Chang, P., and Kosten, T.R. Acupuncture for the treatment of cocaine dependence in methadone-maintained patients. *Am. J. Addict.,* Summer 1993, 2(3): 194–201.

Margolin, A. et al. Effects of real and sham auricular needling: implications for trials of acupuncture for cocaine addiction. *Am. J. Addict.,* 1993, 2(3): 194.

Margolin, A., Chang, P., Avants, S.K., and Kosten, T.R. Effects of sham and real needling: implications for trails of acupuncture for cocaine addiction. *Am. J. Chin. Med.,* 1993, 21(2): 103–111.

Margolin, A. A single-blind investigation of four auricular needle puncture configurations. *Am. J. Chin. Med.,* 1995, 23(2): 105–114.

Marovino, T. Laser auriculotherapy as part of the nicotine detoxification process: evaluation of 1280 subjects and theoretical considerations of a developing model. *Am. J. Acupunc.,* 1994, 22(2): 134.

Martelete, M. Comparative study of analgesic effect of TENS, EAP, and meperidine in treatment of postoperative pain. *Am. J. Acupunc.,* 1986, 14: 168.

Martin, G.P. and Waite, P.M. The efficacy of acupuncture as an aid to stopping smoking. *NZ Med. J.,* Jun. 24, 1981, 93(686): 421–423.

Martina, R.M. How effective is acupuncture without proper detoxification? *Am. J. Acupunc.,* 1989, 17(2): 131–134.

Martynova, G.I., Kurabtseva, O.N., Malyshev, A.V., and Komissarov, V.I. The role of nontraditional methods of analgesia in the post-operative period. *Anesteziol. Reanimatol.,* Mar.–Apr. 1990, 2: 50–51, (in Russian).

Mastroianni, A. The treatment of postoperative pain with the use of semipermanent auricular needles. *Panminerva Med.,* Jan.–Mar. 1985, 27(1): 39–42, (in Italian).

McLellan, A.T., Grossman, D.S., Blaine, J., and Haverkos, H.W. Acupuncture treatment for drug abuse: A technical review. *J. Subst. Abuse Treat.,* Nov.–Dec. 1993, 10(6): 569–576.

Melzack, R. and Katz, J. Auriculotherapy fails to relieve chronic pain: a controlled crossover study. *J. Am. Med. Assoc.,* 1984, 251(8): 1041–1043.

Meng, X.Y. Therapeutic effects of EAP on haemoptysis of pulmonary TB. *Am. J. Acupunc.,* 1986, (Abst) 14: 178, ex *CAP&M,* Feb. 6, 1986: 9–11.

Milani, L. Cases of enuresis nocturna treated with single reflexotherapy. Clinical and therapeutic evaluation. *Minerva Med.,* Nov. 24, 1976, 67(57): 3753–3756, (in Italian).

Milanov, I. and Toteva, S. Acupuncture treatment of tremor in alcohol withdrawal syndrome. *Am. J. Acupunc.,* 1993, 21(4): 319–322.

Mitchell, E.R. *Fighting Drug Abuse with Acupuncture: The Treatment that Works.* Pacific View Press, Berkeley, CA , 1995.

Mitrofanova, N.I., Zagriadskii, V.A., and Durinian, R.A. Auriculotherapy in the treatment of bronchial asthma. *Ter. Arkh.,* 1977, 49(3): 127–129, (in Russian).

Mok M.S., Parker, L.N., Voina, S., and Bray, G.A. Treatment of obesity by acupuncture. *Am. J. Clin. Nutr.,* Aug. 1976, 29(8): 832–835.

Moldovan, C. et al. EAP treatment for superior limb edema, subordinate to radical radiosurgical treatment in patients with mammary neoplasia. *Am. J. Acupunc.,* (Abst.) 1987, 59: 1322.

Moner, S.E. Acupuncture and addiction treatment. *J. Addict. Dis.,* 1996, 15(3): 79–100.

Mu, J. The observation of local analgesic effect of experimental arthritis rats treated with auricular needle. *Chin. Acupunc. Moxibustion,* Oct. 1987, 7(5): 33–35.

Mukaino, Y. Acupuncture therapy for obesity using ear needle treatment: analysis of effectiveness and mechanisms of action. *J. Japn. Soc. Acupres.*, 1981, 31(1): 67–74, (in Japanese).

Mukaino, Y. Effectiveness and mechanism of auricular acupuncture for obesity. *J. Japn. Acupunc. Moxibustion*, 1986, 45(1): 10–25.

Mukhamedzhanov, N.Z., Kurbanova, D.U., and Tahkhodzhaeva, S.I. The principles of the combined rehabilitation of patients with perinatal encephalopathy and its sequelae. *Vopr. Kurortol. Fizioter. Lech. Fiz. Kult.*, Jan.–Feb. 1991, 1: 24–28, (in Russian).

Nakanishi, K., Baron, J.B., Menia, A., Guibret, P., and Grateau, P. Effect of auriculotherapy on vertigo and ataxia due to head injury. *Agressologie*, 1980, 21(E): 157–162, (in French).

Newmeyer, J.A., Johnson, G., and Klot, S. Acupuncture and addiction treatment. *J. Addict. Dis.*, 1996, 15(3): 79–100.

Ng, L.K. Auricular acupuncture in animals: effects of opiate withdrawal and involvement of endorphins. *J. Altern. Comple. Med.*, Spring 1996, 2(1): 61–3; disc. 73–75.

Ng, L.K., Douthitt, T.C., Thoa, N.B., and Albert, C.A. Modification of morphine-withdrawal syndrome in rats following transauricular electrostimulation: an experimental paradigm for auricular electroacupuncture. *Biol. Psych.*, Oct. 1975, 10(5): 575–580.

Ng, L.K., Thoa, N.G., Douthitt, T.C., and Albert, C.A. Experimental auricular electroacupuncture in morphine-dependent rats: behavioral and biochemical observations. *Am. J. Chin. Med.*, Oct. 1975, 3(4): 335–341.

Nezabudkin, S.N., Kachan, A.T., Fedoseev, G.B., and Gamaiunov, K.P. The reflexotherapy of patients with respiratory allergoses. *Ter. Arkh.*, 1992, 64(1): 64–67, (in Russian).

Niu, M. *Functional Bleeding of Uterus with Auriculoacupuncture*. Department of TCM, Dezhou District Hospital, Shendong, China, 1984.

Niu, W.M., Liu, H.Y., and Zhang, Y.H. Application of ear acupuncture therapy to treat opium drug abstinence syndrome. *Shanghai J. Acupunc. Moxibustion*, 2000, 3(6): 27–28.

Noling, L.B., Clelland, J.A., Jackson, J., and Knowles, C. Effects of auricular transcutaneous electrical nerve stimulation on experimental pain threshold. *Phys. Ther.*, Mar. 1988, 68(3): 328–332.

Oliveri, A.C., Clelland, J.A., Jackson, J., and Knowles, C. Effects of auricular transcutaneous electrical nerve stimulation on experimental pain threshold. *Phys. Ther.*, Jan. 1986, 66(1): 1, 2–16.

Olms, J.S. Increased success rate using new acupuncture point for stop smoking discovered. *Am. J. Acupunc.*, Dec. 1984, 12(4): 339–344.

Olms, J.S. New: an effective alcohol abstinence acupuncture treatment. *Am. J. Acupunc.*, 1984, 12(2): 145–148.

Olms, J.S. How to stop smoking: effective new acupuncture point discovered. *Am. J. Acupunc.*, Jul.–Sept. 1981, 9(3): 257–260.

Organ, A.N. The effect of acupuncture on the gastric acid-forming function in patients with duodenal peptic ulcer. *Vopr. Kurortol. Fizioter. Fiz. Kult.*, Sept.–Oct. 1999, 5: 12–14, (in Russian).

Otto, K.C. et al. Auricular acupuncture as an adjunctive treatment for cocaine addiction. A pilot study. *Am. J. Addict.*, 1998, 7(2): 164.

Parker, L.N. and Mok, M.S. The use of acupuncture for smoking withdrawal. *Am. J. Acupunc.*, 1977, 5: 363–366.

Patterson, M.A. Electroacupuncture in alcohol and drug addictions. *Clin. Med.*, 1974, 81(10): 9–13.

Patterson, M. *Addictions Can Be Cured. The Treatment of Drug Addiction by Neuro-electric Stimulation: An Interim Report*, 1st ed. Lion Press, Berkhamsted, U.K., 1975.

Peng, Y., Fenglan, L., and Xin, W. Treatment of essential hypertension with auriculopressure. *J. Trad. Chin. Med.*, 1991, 1117–1121.

Peng, X.C. Stop smoking by acupoint sticking therapy. Short-term follow-up studies of 126 cases. *Chin. Acupunc. Moxibustion*, 1984, 4(1): 7.

Pert, A., Dionne, R., Ng, L., Bragin, E., Moody, T.W., and Pert, C. Alteration in rat central nervous system endorphins following transauricular electroacupuncture. *Brain Res.*, 1981, 224(1): 83–93.

Pesikov, I.S. New method of ear acupuncture in the treatment of chronic and protracted diseases. *Ter. Arkh.*, 1982, 54(1): 114–116, (in Russian).

Pilloni, C., Caracausi, R.S., Tognali, F., and Sbarbaro, V. EEG evaluation of patients undergoing extracorporeal circulation under analgesic and electrohyoalgesia with auricular acupuncture. *Minerva Anestesiol.*, Mar. 1980, 46(3): 371–386, (in Italian).

Pontinin, P.M. Long-term experiences in the treatment of obesity by implanted ear press needles in hypertensive patients. *Acupunc. Electrother. Res.*, 1985, 10(3): 211–212.

Privitera, P. Vertigo and auriculotherapy. *Minerva Med.*, Mar. 31, 1980, 71(12): 931–933, (in Italian).

Privitera, P. Auriculotherapy and pneumarthrocentesis in the treatment of hydrarthrosis of the knee. *Minerva Med.*, Nov. 17, 1977, 68(56): 3804–3805, (in Italian).

Qin, G.F. 413 cases of abnormal fetal position corrected by auricular plaster therapy. *J. Trad. Chin. Med.*, Dec. 1989, 9(4): 235–237.

Qin, X.L. Observation of the therapeutic effect of 130 cases of abdominal pain by EAP at GV11 and GV09. *AJA*, (Abst.), 1988, 16:180, ex *CAP&M*, Dec. 1987, 7: 25.

Rabl, V., Bochdansky, T., Hertz, H., Kern, H., and Meng, A. The effect of standardized acupuncture programs in the after-care of accident patients. *Unfallchirurgie*, Dec. 1983, 9(6): 308–313, (in German).

Radzievskii, S.A., and Vorontsova, E.L. The effect of electroacupuncture and acupuncture on ischemic and reperfusion cardiac arrhythmias. *Vopr. Kurortol. Fizioter. Lech. Fiz. Kult.*, Nov.–Dec. 1989, 6: 7–9, (in Russian).

Rampes, H., Pereira, S., Mortimer, A., Manoharan, S., and Knowles, M. Does electroacupuncture reduce craving for alcohol? A randomized controlled study. *Compli. Ther. Med.*, 1997, 5(1): 19–26.

Rampes, H. and Pereira, S. Role of acupuncture in alcohol dependence and abuse. *Acupunc. Med.*, Nov. 1993, 11(2): 80–84.

Raevskaia, O.S. Nocioceptive sensitivity of rabbits in varying localization of pain stimuli and naloxone administration. *Patol. Fiziol. Eksp. Ter.*, Sept.–Dec. 1992, 5–6: 7–9.

Requena, Y., Michel, D., Fabre, J., Pernice, C., and Nguyen, J. Smoking withdrawal therapy by acupuncture. *Am. J. Acupunc.*, 1980, 8(1): 57–63.

Richard, A.J., Montoya, I.D., Nelson, R., and Spence, R.T. Effectiveness of adjunct therapies in crack cocaine treatment. *J. Subst. Abuse Treat.*, Nov.–Dec. 1995, 12(6): 401–413.

Richards, D. and Marley, J. Stimulation of auricular points in weight loss. *Aust. Fam. Phys.*, Jul., 27, 1998, (Suppl.) 2: S 73–77.

Riet, G.T., Kleijnen, P., and Knipschild, P. A meta-analysis of studies into the effect of acupuncture on addiction. *Br. J. Gen. Pract.*, 1990, 40(338): 379–382.

Romoli, M. and Giommi, A. Ear acupuncture and psychosomatic medicine: right-left asymmetry of acupoints and lateral preferences – Part II. *Acupunc. Electrother. Res.*, Jan.–Mar. 1994, 19(1): 11–17.

Romoli, M. and Giommi, A. Ear acupuncture in psychosomatic medicine; the importance of the Sanjiao (triple heater) area. *Acupunc. Electrother. Res.*, 1993 Jul.–Dec., 18(3–4): 185–194.

Romoli, M., Tordini, G., and Giommi, A. Diagonal ear-lobe crease: possible significance as cardiovascular risk factor and its relationship to ear-acupuncture. *Acupunc. Electrother. Res.*, 1989, 14(2): 149–154.

Romoli, M., van der Windt, D., Giovanzana, P., Masserano, G., Vignali, F., Quirico, E., and Giommi, A. International research project to devise a protocol to test the effectiveness of acupuncture on painful shoulder. *J. Altern. Comple. Med.*, Jun. 2000, 6(3): 281–287.

Rongxing, Z., Yanhua, Z., and Lu, Y. Hypotensive effect of ototherapy in relation to symptomatic and dispositional types of patients. *J. Trad. Chin. Med.*, 1992, 12: 124–128.

Rongxing, Z., Yanhua, Z., Jialiang, W., Hong, C., and Jian, F. Antihypertensive effect of auriculo-acupoint pressing therapy – clinical analysis of cases. *J. Trad. Chin. Med.*, 1991, 11: 89–92.

Rossano, N.A. Crack-cocaine abuse acupuncture as effective adjunct to therapy in current treatment programs. *Int. J. Clin. Acupunc.*, 1992, 3(4): 333–338.

Russell, L.C., Sharp, B., and Gilbertson, B. Acupuncture for addicted patients with chronic histories of arrest. A pilot study of the Consortium Treatment Center. *J. Sub. Abuse Treat.*, Sept. 2000, 19(2): 199–205.

Roustan, C. Alcoolisme et acupuncture. *Rev. Fr. Acupunc.*, 1992, 18(72): 11–19, (in French).

Sacks, L.L. Drug addiction: alcoholism, smoking, and obesity treated by auricular staplepuncture. *Am. J. Acupunc.*, 1975, 3(2): 147–150.

Sainsbury, M.J. Acupuncture in heroin withdrawal. *Med. J. Aust.*, Jul. 20, 1974, 2(3): 102–105.

Sainsbury, M.J. Heroin withdrawal using ear acupuncture. *Med. J. Aust.*, Jun. 1974, 1(22): 899.

Saku, K., Mukaino, Y., Ying, H., and Arakawa, K. Characteristics of reactive electropermeable points on the auricles of coronary heart disease patients. *Clin. Cardio.*, May 1993, 16(5): 415–419.

Sapir–Weise, R., Berglund, M., and Kristenson, H. Acupuncture in alcoholism treatment: a randomized out-patient study. *Alcoh. Alcoh.*, Jul.–Aug. 1999, 34(4): 629–635.

Scherkovina, T.I. and Gaponiuk, P.I. Effect of auricular acupuncture therapy on central hemodynamics in patients with hypertension. *Vopr. Kurortol. Fizioter. Lech. Fiz. Kult.*, Jan.–Feb. 1998, 1: 20–22, (in Russian).

Schwartz, J.L. Evaluation of acupuncture as a treatment for smoking. *Am. J. Acupunc.*, 1988, 16(2): 135–142.

Sedlacek, P.R., Clelland, J.A., Knowles, C., Jackson, J.R., and Varner, R.E. Jr. Electrical conductance at auricular acupuncture points during dysmenorrhea. *Clin. J. Pain*, 1988, 4(3): 183–190.

Selacek, P. et al. Electrical conductance at auricular acupuncture points during dysmenorrhea. *Clin. J. Pain*, 1988, 4: 183–190.

Serizawa, K. *Clinical Acupuncture, A Practical Japanese Approach*. Japan Publications, Tokyo, 1988.

Seversen, L., Markoff, R.A., and Chun–Hoo, A. Heroin detox with acupuncture and electrical stimulation. *Int. J. Addict.*, 1977, 12(7): 911–922.

Shafshak, T.S. Electroacupuncture and exercise in body weight reduction and their application in rehabilitating patients with knee osteoarthritis. *Am. J. Chin. Med.*, 1995, 23(1): 15–25.

Shakar, M. and Smith, M. The use of acupuncture in the treatment of drug addiction. *Am. J. Acupunc.*, Jul.–Sept. 1979, 7(3): 223–228.

Shanghai Medical School Acupuncture Study Group. Auricular acupuncture on smoking taste and plasma endorphins. *Shanghai J. Acupunc. Moxibustion*, 1985, 1–3.

Shapiro, R.S., Christopher, W., and Cicora, B. Effective stimulation of auricular and body acupuncture materials. *Vet. Acupunc. Newsl.*, Jan.–Mar. 1989, 14(1): 25–36.

Shi, Z.X. Observation on the curative effect of 120 cases of auditory hallucination treated with auricular acupuncture. *J. Trad. Chin. Med.*, Sept. 1998, 9(3): 176–178.

Shiraishi, T., Onoe, M., Kageyyama, T., Sameshima, Y., Kojima, T., Konishi, S., Yoshimatsu, H., and Sakata, T. Effects of auricular acupuncture on nonobese, healthy volunteer subjects. *Obes. Res.*, Dec. 1995, 3 (Suppl.) 5: 6673–6676.

Shiraishi, T., Onoe, M., Kojima, T., Sameshima, Y., and Kageyama, T. Effects of auricular stimulation on feeding-related hypothalamic neuronal activity in normal and obese rats. *Brain Res. Bull.*, 1995, 36(2): 141–148.

Shulan, L. 47 cases of severe hiccup treated by auricular acupuncture. *Chin. J. Acupunc. Moxibustion*, 1990, 3(1): 55–56.

Simmons, M.S. and Oleson, T.D. Auricular electrical stimulation and dental pain threshold. *Anesth. Prog.*, 1993, 40(1): 14–19.

Smirala, J. Ear acupuncture and its use in anesthesiology. *Bratisl. Lek. Listy.*, May 1978, 69(5): 612–619, (in Slovak).

Smith, M.O., Aponte, J., Bonilla–Rodriguez, R., Rabinowitz, N., Cintron, F., and Hernandez, L. Acupuncture detoxification in a drug and alcohol abuse treatment setting. *Am. J. Acupunc.*, 1984, 12(3): 251–255.

Smith, M.O. and Khan, I. An acupuncture program for the treatment of drug-addicted persons. *Bull. Narc.*, 1988, 40(1): 35–41.

Smith, M.O. Acupuncture and natural healing in drug detoxification. *Am. J. Acupunc.*, Apr.–Jun. 1979, 7(2): 97–107.

Smith, M.O. Acupuncture treatment for crack: clinical survey of 1500 patients treated. *Am. J. Acupunc.*, 1988, 16(3): 241–246.

Smith, M.O., Sqires, R., Aponte, J., Rabinovits, N., and Bonilla–Rodriguez, R. Acupuncture treatment of drug addiction and alcohol abuse. *Am. J. Acupunc.*, Jun. 1982, 10(2): 161–166.

Smith, M.O. and Khan, I. An acupuncture program for the treatment of drug-addicted persons. *Bull. Narc.*, 1988, 40(1): 35–41.

Smith, M.O. Acupuncture treatment of drug addiction and alcohol abuse. *J. Trad. Chin. Med.*, Dec. 1988, 8(4): 263–264.

Solun, M.N. and Liaifer, A.L. Acupuncture in the treatment of diabetic angiopathy of the lower extremities. *Probl. Endokrinol.* (Mosk.), Jul.–Aug. 1991, 37(4): 20–23, (in Russian).

Song, G.Y. 100 Cases of mumps treated with ear needling on Pingjian point (MA– T 2). *J. Trad. Chin. Med.*, 1989, 9(1): 14.

Soong, S.Y. The treatment of exogenous obesity employing auricular acupuncture. *Am. J. Acupunc.*, 1975, 3(3): 285–287.

Southall, D. Complementary therapy to fight drug addiction. *Nurs. Times.*, Aug. 13–19, 1977, 93(33): 48–49.

Spacek, A., Huemer, G., Grubhofer, G., Lackner, F.X., Zwolfer, W., and Kress, H.G. The use of ear acupuncture (P29–PAD, Occiput) in the case of a drop in blood pressure following the administration of Thiopental. *Dtsch. Z. Akupunkt.*, 1996, 39(1): 18–22, (in German).

Spears, C. Auricular acupuncture; new approach to treatment of cerebral palsy. *Am. J. Acupunc.*, Jan.–Mar. 1979, 1(7): 49–54.

Spoerel, W.É., Varkey, M., and Leung, C. Acupuncture in chronic pain. *Am. J. Chin. Med.*, Autumn 1976, 4(3): 267–279.

Steiner, R.P., Hay, D.L., and Davis, A.W. Acupuncture therapy for the treatment of tobacco smoking addiction. *Am. J. Chin. Med.*, 1982, 10(1–4): 107–121.

Still, J. Auriculotherapy and canine thoracolumbar disc disease. *J. S. Afr. Vet. Assoc.*, Mar. 1992, 62(1): 3.

Still, J. A clinical study of auriculotherapy in canine thoracolumbar discs disease. *J. S. Afr. Vet. Assoc.*, Sept. 1990, 61(3): 102–105.

Strom, H. Effect of electro-acupuncture of the ear on joint movement and pain after meniscectomy. A controlled triple-blind study. *Ugeskr. Laeger.*, Sept. 26, 1977, 139(30): 2326–2329, (in Danish).

Sun, E.L. Weight reduction with auricular acupuncture. *Am. J. Acupunc.*, Oct.–Dec. 1979, 7(4): 311–355.

Sun, H. Clinical observation on auricular acupuncture for treatment of pain diseases. Am. *J. Trad. Chin. Med.*, 2001, 2(1): 15–17.

Sun, Q. Simple obesity and hyperlipidemia treated with otopoint pellet pressure and body acupuncture. *J. Trad. Chin. Med.*, Mar. 1993, 13(1): 22–26.

Sun, S.H. et al. Stop smoking treated by ear acupuncture. *Chin. Acupunc. Moxibustion*, Oct. 1986, 6(5): 4, (in Chinese).

Sytinsky, I.A., Galebskaya, L.V., and Jantunen, A. Physiologo-biochemical basis of drug dependence treatment by electroacupuncture. *Am. J. Acupunc.*, 1981, 1(9).

Tabeeva, D.M. and Akhtiamov, I.S. Effect of auricular acupuncture on the organization of night sleep. *Klin. Med.* (Mosk.), Oct. 1980, 58(10): 102–105, (in Russian).

Tabeeva, D.M. Autonomic nervous system function of alcoholics during acupuncture treatment. *ZH Nevropatol. Psikhiatr. IM. S.S. Korsakova*, 1988, 88(10): 33–36, (in Russian).

Tabeeva, D.M. and Shagieva, L.K. Comparative analysis of the efficacy of different methods of acupuncture in the hyper-and hypokinetic types of circulation in hypertensive patients. *ZH Nevropatol. Psikhiatr. IM S.S. Korsakova*, 1984, 84(1): 47–50, (in Russian).

Tan, Y. Clinical observation of the treatment of cigarette smoking by implanted auricular acupuncture. 1988, *Proceedings of 4th International Congress of Chinese Medicine*, 14.

Tanaka, O. The effect of auricular acupuncture on olfactory acuity. *Am. J. Chin. Med.*, 1999, 27(1): 19–24.

Tang, X. 75 cases of simple obesity treated with auricular and body acupuncture. *J. Trad. Chin. Med.*, Mar. 1997, 17(1): 55–56.

Tekeoglu, I., Adak, B., and Ercan, M. Investigation into the possibilities of using ear acupressure for increasing the pain threshold during athletic training. *Am. J. Acupunc.*, 26 (1): 49–52.

Tennant, F.S. Jr. Outpatient heroin detoxification with acupuncture and staplepuncture. *West J. Med.*, Sept. 1976, 125(3): 191–194.

Ter Riet, G., Kleijnen, J., and Knipschild, P. A meta-analysis of studies into the effect of acupuncture on addiction. *Br. J. Gen. Pract.*, Sept. 1990, 40 (338): 379–382.

Thorer, H. and Volf, N. Acupuncture after alcohol consumption: A sham controlled assessment. *Acupunc. Med.*, 1996, 14(2): 63–67.

Tian, L. Composite acupuncture treatment of mental retardation in children. *J. Trad. Chin. Med.*, Mar. 1995, 15(3): 34–37.

Tian, Z.M. and Chu, Y.W. Treating smoking addiction with the ear point seed pressing method. *J. Chin. Med.*, Sept. 1996, 52: 5–6.

Tian, L. Composite acupuncture treatment of mental retardation in children. *J. Trad. Chin. Med.*, 1995 Mar., 15(3): 34–37.

Timofeev, M.F. Effects of acupuncture and an antagonist of opiate receptors on heroin dependent patients. *Am. J. Chin. Med.*, 1999, 27(2): 143–148.

Torre, L. Lumbosciatic and Nogier's auriculotherapy: consideration of 50 cases. *Minerva Med.*, 1979, 67(5): 356–358.

Toteva, S. and Milanov, I. The use of body acupuncture for treatment of alcohol dependence and withdrawal syndrome: a controlled study. *Am. J. Acupunc.*, 1996, 24(1): 19–25.

Troshin, O.V. The functional properties of the cochlear vestibular points of the external auditory canal. *Fiziol. ZH*, Mar. 1993, 79(3): 47–53, (in Russian).

Umeh, B. Ear acupuncture using semi-permanent needles: acceptability, prospects, and problems in Nigeria. *Am. J. Acupunc.*, 1988, 16 (1–2): 67–70.

Voteva, S. Use of body acupuncture for treatment of alcohol dependence and withdrawal syndrome. *Am. J. Acupunc.*, 1996, 24(1): 19–25.

Vandevenne, A., Rempp, M., Burghard, G. et al. Study of the specific contribution of acupuncture to tobacco detoxification. *Sem. Hop.*, 1985, 61(29): 2155–2160, (in French).

Vashchenko, E.A., Garkavenko, V.V., Limanskii, I.P., and Lipko, I.B. Effect of electric stimulation of auricular acupuncture points on H–reflex. *Fiziol. ZH*, Nov.–Dec. 1989, 35(6): 88–91, (in Russian).

Vasilenko, A.M., Kirilina, E.A., and Sarybaeva, D.V. Prevention and correction of stress-induced immunodeficiency by atrial electroacupuncture. *Patol. Fisiol. Eksp. Ter.*, May–Jun. 1989, 3: 21–24, (in Russian).

Vatanparast, Z., Watzak, M., Spacek, A., and Zwolfer, W. Ear acupuncture combined with dietetic consultation for the purpose of weight reduction. *Dtsch. Z. Akupunkt.*, 1995, 38(4):95–99, (in German).

Visetti, E. and Costa, P. Auriculotherapy for intra-operative hiccup in anesthetized patients. *Am. J. Acupunc.*, 1995, 23(2): 105–108.

Vozainov, A.F., Paeechnikov, S.P., and Kovtuniak, O.N. The laser reflexotherapy of patients with chronic prostatitis. *Vrach. Delo.*, Feb. 1991, 2: 45–48, (in Russian).

Waite, N.R. and Clough, J.B. A single-blind, placebo-controlled trial of a simple acupuncture treatment in the cessation of smoking. *Br. J. Gen. Prac.*, 1998, 48(433): 1487–1490.

Wang, F.H., Chen, C.L., Chen, M.C., Wang, P.Y., Lin, J.M., and Jih, K.S. Auricular electroacupuncture for postthoracotomy pain. *Zhonghua Yi Xue Za Zhi*, May 1988, 41(5): 349–356, (in Chinese).

Wang, M.L. 42 cases of climacteric syndrome treated with auricular pellet pressure. *J. Trad. Chin. Med*, Sept. 1991, 11(3): 196–198.

Wang, Q. and Zhao, Y.Y. Treatment of urinary retention due to post-operative anal pain. *J. Trad. Chin. Med.*, Sept. 1991, 11(3): 199–200.

Wang, R.Z. Introduction to auricular point sticking to stop smoking. Shaanxi *J. Chin. Trad. Med.*, 1989, 10(1): 31, (in Chinese).

Wang, S.M. and Kain, Z.N. Auricular acupuncture: a potential treatment for anxiety. *Anesth. Analg.*, Feb. 2001, 92(2): 548–553.

Wang, T. Auricular acupoint pellet pressure in the treatment of cholelithiasis, *J. Trad. Chin. Med.*, Jun. 1990, 10(2): 126–131.

Wang, X.M. Therapeutic effect of EAP with moxa in 95 cases of chronic pelvic inflammatory disease. *Am. J. Acupunc.*, 1989, (Abst.) 17: 275–276; ex *JTCM* 1989, 9/1: 21–24.

Wang, X.M. Analysis of therapeutic effects in 110 cases of intestinal adhesion treated by EAP. *Am. J. Acupunc.*, 1987, 15: 270.

Wang, Y.X. Observation on the effect of 303 cases of liver and gallstone treatment of ear point pressure. *Chin. Acupunc. Moxibustion,* 1989, 9(1): 8, (in Chinese).

Wang, Z. and Wang, J. 200 Cases of oticodina treated by auricular point pressing therapy. *Chin. Acupunc. Moxibustion*, 1991, 4(2): 112–114.

Washburn, A.M. et al. Acupuncture heroin detoxification: a single-blind clinical trial. *J. Subst. Abuse*, 10(4): 345, 1993.

Washburn, A.M., Fullilove, R.E., Fullilove, M.T., Keenan, P.A., McGee, B., Morris, K.A., Sorensen, J.L., and Clark, W.W. Acupuncture heroin detoxification: a single-blind clinical trial. *J. Subst. Abuse Treat.*, Jul.–Aug. 1993, 10(4): 345–351.

Wells, E.A., Jackson, R., Diaz, O.R., Stanton, V., Saxon, A.J., and Krupski, A. Acupuncture as an adjunct to methadone treatment services. *Am. J. Addict.*, 1995, 4(3): 198–214.

Wen, H. and Teo, S.W. Experience in the treatment of drug addiction by electroacupuncture. *Mod. Med. Asia*, Jun. 1975, 11(6): 23–24.

Wen, H.L. and Cheung, S.Y. How acupuncture can help addicts. *Drugs Society*, 1973, 2: 18–20.

Wen, H.L. and Cheung, S.Y.C. Treatment of drug addiction by acupuncture and electrical stimulation. *Am. J. Acupunc.*, Apr.–Jun. 1973, 1: 71–75.

Wen, H.L. and Cheung, Y.C. Treatment of drug addiction by acupuncture and electrical stimulation, *Asian J. Med.*, 1973, 9: 138.

Wen, H.L., Ho, W.K., Wong, H.K., Hehal, Z.D., Ng, Y.H., and Ma, L. Changes in adrenocorticotropic hormone (ACTH) and cortisol in drug addicts treated by acupuncture and electrical stimulation (AES). *Comp. Med. East West*, 1979, 6(1): 61–66.

Wen, H.L., Ng, Y.H., Ho, W.K., Fung, K.P., Wong, H.K., Ma, L., and Wong, H.C. Acupuncture in narcotic withdrawal: A preliminary report on biochemical changes in the blood and urine of heroin addicts. *Bull. Narc.*, Apr.–Jun. 1978, 30(2): 31–39.

Wen, H.L. Acupuncture and electrical stimulation (AES) outpatient detoxification. *Mod. Med. Asia*, Jun. 1975, 11(6): 23–24.

Wen, H.L. and Cheung, A.Y.C. Treatment of drug addiction by acupuncture and electrical stimulation. *Am. J. Acupunc.*, 1973, 1(2): 71–75.

Wen, H.L. Clinical experience and mechanism of acupuncture and electrical stimulation (AES) in the treatment of drug abuse. *Am. J. Chin. Med.*, 1980, 8(4): 349–353.

Wen, H.L. Fast detoxification of heroin addicts by acupuncture and electrical stimulation (AES) in combination with naloxone. *Comp. Med. East West*, Fall–Winter 1977, 5(3–4): 257–263.

White A.R. and Rampes, H. Acupuncture in smoking cessation. *Cochran Database Sys. Rev.*, 2000, 2: CD000009.

World Congress of Medical Acupuncture, Edmonton, Alberta. Possible new treatment of Parkinson's by auriculotherapy, 1995.

Worner, T.M., Zeller, B., Schwarz, H., Zwas, F., and Lyon, D. Acupuncture fails to improve treatment outcome in alcoholics. *Drug Alc. Depend.*, Jun. 1992, 30(2): 169–173.

Wu, H., Bi, L., Xu, C., and Zhu, P. Analgesic effect of pressure on auriculoacupoints for post operative pain in 102 cases. *J. Chin. Med.*, Mar. 1991, 11(1): 22–25.

Wu, H.P., Bi, L.Y., Xu, C.S., and Zhu, P.T. Clinical observation of 50 cases of postoperative incisional pain treated by auricular-acupoint pressure. *J. Trad. Chin. Med.*, Sept. 1989, 9(3): 187–189.

Wu, H. et al. Clinical observation and mechanism study in application of auricular-pressing pill for post-operative analgesia. *J. Trad. Chin. Med.*, 1991, 17(1): 26–31.

Wu, Y. The effect of acupuncture in curing the smoking habit, 210 cases. *J. Trad. Chin. Med.*, 1981, 1(1): 65–66.

Wu, Y. Treatment of acute pain with auricular pellet pressure on ear Shenmen as main point. *J. Trad. Chin. Med.*, Jun. 1992, 12(2): 114–115.

Wu, Y.L. et al. Relationship between central cholinergic activity and pressor effect of EAP. 2.: under hypotension. *Am. J. Acupunc.*, 1984, 12: 383–384, ex *CAP&M*, Jun. 1984, 4: 34–37.

Wu, Y.X. Treatment of 32 cases of pseudobulbar palsy by EAP, *Abstract AJA*, 1984, 12: 386, ex *CAP&M*, 1984, 4(1): 10–11.

Xiaoming, M., Ling, L., Yunxing, P., Guifang, X., et al. Clinical studies on the mechanism for acupuncture stimulation of ovulation. *J. Trad. Chin. Med.*, 1993, 13: 115–119.

Xu, B. Clinical observation of the weight reducing effect of ear acupuncture in 350 cases of obesity. *J. Trad. Chin. Med.*, 1985, 5(2): 87–88.

Xu, Y.H. Treatment of acne with ear acupuncture – a clinical observation of 80 cases. *J. Trad. Chin. Med.*, Dec. 1989, 9(4): 238–239.

Xu, G.S. and Liu, W.Z. Double phasic modulatory effects of auricular point electroacupuncture on gastrointestinal electric activity in rabbits. *Zhong Xi Yi Jie He Za Zhi*, Nov. 1988, 8(11): 671–673, 646, (in Chinese).

Xudong, G. Clinical study on analgesia for biliary colic with ear acupuncture at point Erzhong. *Am. J. Acupunc.*, 1993, 21(3): 237–239.

Yan, S. 14 cases of child bronchial asthma treatment by auricular plaster and meridian instrument. *J. Trad. Chin. Med.*, Sept. 1998, 18(3): 202–204.

Yang, C. et al. 268 cases of myopia treated with injection and pellet pressure at auriculopoints. *J. Trad. Chin. Med.*, Sept. 1993., 13(3): 196–198.

Yang, C.L. Clinical observation of 62 cases of insomnia treated by auricular point imbedding therapy. *J. Trad. Chin. Med.*, Sept. 1988, 8(3): 190–192.

Yang, C.L. Treatment of 1040 cases of myopia with auriculotherapy using medicated pellets. *J. Trad. Chin. Med.*, Dec. 1987, 7(4): 273–278.

Yang, M.M. and Kwok, J.S. Evaluation on the treatment of morphine addiction by acupuncture Chinese herbs and opioid peptides. *Am. J. Chin. Med.*, 1986, 14(1–2): 46–50.

Yang, R. and Fang, H.W. Use of acupuncture on the ear points "xia ping gian" and "xia jiao gou" to induce blood pressure changes. Paper presented at the 4th International Congress of Chinese Medicine, University of San Francisco, CA, Jul. 29–31, 1988.

Yao, S. 46 cases of insomnia treated by semicondictor laser irradiation on auricular points. *J. Trad. Chin. Med.*, Dec. 1999, 19(4): 298–299.

Yihou, X. Treatment of acne with ear acupuncture – a clinical observation of 80 cases. *J. Trad. Chin. Med.*, 1989, 9: 238–239.

Yu, J., Huang, W.Y., and Zheng, H.M. EAP induced ovulation and changes in skin temperature of the hand. *Am. J. Acupunc.*, 1987, (Abst.) 15: 276–277, ex *CJIT & WM*, 1986, 6: 720–722.

Zalesskiy, V.N., Belousova, I.A., and Frolov, G.V. Laser-acupuncture reduces cigarette smoking: a preliminary report. *Acupunc. Electrother. Res.*, 1983, 8(3–4): 297–302.

Zhan, J. Observations on the treatment of 393 cases of obesity by semen pressure on auricular points. *J. Trad. Chin. Med.*, Mar. 1993, 13(1): 27–30.

Zhang, J.M., Tan, S.G., and Yu, J.S. Stop smoking by auricular acupoint sticking therapy combined with Chinese herbal drug pressure at body acupoints. Report of 120 cases. Shaanxi Correspond. *J. Trad. Chin. Med.*, 1989, (4): 28–29, (in Chinese).

Zhang, C.C. The endogenous opiate and nonopiate analgesic system. *Zhen Ci Yan Jiu*, 1989, 149: 306–314, (in Chinese).

Zhang, L. Alcoholic abstinence by electroacupuncture plus auriculo-pressure in 18 cases. *TCM Shanghai J. Acupunc. Moxibustion*, 2001, 4(1): 64–65.

Zhang, L.C. Treatment of myopia with ear-point pressing and acupuncture: a report of 216 cases. *Int. J. Clin. Acupunc.*, 1995, 6(1): 105–107.

Zhang, R. The effect of auricular-plaster therapy on gallstone expulsion and on expansion-contraction function of the biliary system – a clinical analysis of 57 cases. *J. Trad. Chin. Med.*, Dec. 1986, 6(4): 262–266.

Zhang, Y., Li, Y., Tang, X., Ji, C., and Chen, L. The effect of stimulating auricular liver-gall point on the size of a gallbladder of the rabbit. *Zhen Ci Yan Jiu*, 1993, 18(1): 73–74, (in Chinese).

Zhang, Z. Weight reduction by auriculo-acupuncture – a report of 110 cases. *J. Trad. Chin. Med.*, Mar. 1990, 10(1): 17–18.

Zhao, C. Treatment of acute cerebro-vascular diseases and sequelae with acupuncture. *J. Trad. Chin. Med.*, Mar. 1990, 10(1): 70–73.

Zhao, C.X. Acupuncture treatment of morning sickness. *J. Trad. Chin. Med.*, Sept. 1988, 8(3): 228–229.

Zhao, C.X. Acupuncture and moxibustion treatment of hiccup. *J. Trad. Chin. Med.*, Sept. 1988, 9(3): 182–183.

Zhao, S. Infant fever treated by auricular therapy. *Chin. Acupunc. Moxibustion*, 1985, 5(4): 13–14.

Zhou, R.X., Zhang, Y.H., et al. Anti-hypertensive effect of auriculo-acupoint pressing therapy – clinical analysis of 274 cases. *J. Trad. Chin. Med.*, 1991, 11(1): 189–192.

Zhou, L. and Chey, W.Y. Subcutaneous EAP causes non-parietal cell secretion of the stomach in dogs. *AJA*, 1983, (Abst.) 11: 280–281; ex *Gastroenterology*, 1983, 84: 1359 (meeting paper abstract).

Zhou, R., Zhang, Y., and Ye, L. Hypotensive effect of ototherapy in relation to symptomatic and dispositional types of patients. *J. Trad. Chin. Med.*, Jun. 1992, 12(2): 134–138.

Zhou, R.X., Zhang, Y.H., et al. Anti-hypertensive effect of auriculo-acupoint pressing therapy – clinical analysis of 274 cases. *J. Trad. Chin. Med.*, 1991, 11(1): 189–192.

Zhu, B., Wang, Y., and Xu, W. Effect of electroacupuncture on peripheral microcirculation in acute experimental arthritic rats. *Zhen Ci Yan Jiu*, 1993, 18(3): 219–222, (in Chinese).

Zhunqin, G. Review on the experimental research on auricular points and their diagnostic and therapeutic mechanism. *Int. J. Clin. Acupunc.*, 2001, 12(3): 265–276.

Zudong, G. Clinical study on analgesia for biliary colic with ear acupuncture at point Erzhong. *Am. J. Acupunc.*, 1993, 21(3): 237–239.

Conclusion

This brief synopsis of many areas applicable to auricular medicine can provide the reader with a sense of research done in the field as well as its clinical success. With ear acupuncture, almost every illness can benefit from its use.

As I have mentioned, this book was not meant to be a treatment of disease text nor to list or reconcile the various ear maps that have been generated over the years. These books abound. Rather, the ability to think about how to use a point based upon its traditional Chinese energetics will empower the practitioner to select these 100 simple points in order to help many, many patients. Familiarity with point locations, contraindications, modalities, and prescription writing along with the skill to diagnose and differentiate disease will lead to the successful utilization of auricular medicine for either the prevention of illness or its direct treatment.

In the hundreds of simple and oftentimes emergency treatments that I have administered I have certainly been humbled by the profound power of the ear accessed through the tools of Chinese auricular medicine, many times simply through the power of touch of the human hand to the ear.

Today there are many tools available to a healthcare practitioner in any tradition that can be chosen for their curative effect as well as the comfort that they bestow. But in my experience few rival the unprecedented power of energy encapsulated in the miraculous orifice of the ear that are part of the treatment repertoire of Chinese medicine. So practice with diagnostic acumen and compassion and glean your own clinical experience and you will help many people living in suffering and disharmony through the simple treatment of the ear which continues to play a profound role in culture, physiology and the healing of the human condition.

French acupuncturist Paul Nogier wisely said, "Each doctor needs to be convinced of the efficacy of this ear reflex method by personal results that he or she is right. They are indeed fortunate people who can convince themselves simply by noting the improvement of a symptom they themselves have experienced."

The ear plays a rich role in culture and medicine. So glean your own experience, and you will help many people living in suffering and disharmony.

Appendix A: Definition of Terms

Ancestral energy Prenatal *Qi*, *Yuan Qi*, the original *Qi* one acquires from one's parents, genetic inheritance

Blood The Chinese conception of blood that consists of body fluids (*Jinye*), Nutritive *Qi*, and Essence of the Kidney (*Jing*)

Channels and collaterals The meridians and the *Luo* vessels respectively that run throughout the body and contain *Qi* and Blood

Da Qi The sensation of the arrival of *Qi* to the needle

Endogenous pathogens The emotions

Essence *Jing*, a rarefied form of stored *Qi*

Essential substances The building blocks of life according to Chinese medicine — *Qi*, Blood, *Jing*, *Jinye* (Body fluids), *Shen*, and *Marrow*

Exogenous pathogens The external climates or other factors that mimic the external climates, such as Wind, Cold, Damp, Dryness, Heat or Summer Heat, or a combination of these

***Fu* organs** The six *Yang* or hollow organs

Jiao Heater, warmer, burning space as in the *Sanjiao*

Jing Rarefied essence, one of the essential substances

Neijing The oldest body of Chinese medical literature, about 500 to 300 B.C., also referred to as The Canon of Acupuncture, The Compendium of Acupuncture and Moxibustion, The Yellow Emperor's Classic, and The Classic of Internal Medicine

Organ-meridian complex The Chinese concept of organ, which is not the gross anatomical organ per se, but the entire organ/energetic (physiological) sphere of function that it encompasses in Oriental medicine

Phlegm A secondary pathological product in Oriental medicine, somewhat analogous to phlegm in Western medicine

Qi Vital energy or life force, the primary physical construct of Oriental medicine that explains most physiological processes

Sanjiao The Triple Warmer, the three *jiaos* or sections of the body

The Three Treasures A particular diagnostic framework referring to *Jing, Qi,* and *Shen*

Wei Qi Protective, defensive *Qi*

Ying Qi Nutritive energy

Zang The six *Yin* or solid organs

Zang-fu The 12 organs in Oriental medicine

- For reader convenience, all Chinese terms are italicized
- To distinguish the western concept of organ from the Chinese concept of organ, the Chinese organ-meridian complex is capitalized, i.e., lung vs. Lung

Appendix B: Suppliers and Associations

Suppliers

Helio Medical Supplies, Inc.
606 Charcot Avenue
San Jose, CA 95131
Phone: 408-433-3355
Fax: 408-433-5566

Lhasa Medical, Inc.
234 Libbey Parkway
Weymouth, MA 02189
Phone: 800-722-8775
Fax: 781-335-6296
www.LhasaMedical.com

Oriental Medical Suppliers (OMS)
1950 Washington Street
Braintree, MA 02185
Phone: 800-323-1839
Fax: 781-335-5779
www.omsmedical.com

Associations

Auriculotherapy International Research and Training Center
2905 Lakeview Drive
Fern Park, FL 32730
Phone: 407-830-0068
Fax: 407-830-5044

Groupe Lyonnais d'Etudes Medicales (GLEM)/Nogier website
49 Rue Merciere 69002
Lyon, France
Phone: 0-472-414008
Fax: 0-487-375514

Society of Auricular Acupuncturists
Nurstead Lodge
Nurstead Church Lane, Meopham
Kent DA13 9AD, U.K.
Phone/Fax: 01474 813902

Index

D

E

J

K

L

M

N

S

T

U

V

W